Atlas of Feline Ophthalmology

Atlas of Feline Ophthalmology

Second Edition

Kerry L. Ketring, DVM
Diplomate, ACVO
All Animal Eye Clinic
Whitehall, Michigan

Mary Belle Glaze, DVM, MS
Diplomate, ACVO
Gulf Coast Animal Eye Clinic
Houston, Texas

(W) WILEY-BLACKWELL
A John Wiley & Sons, Ltd., Publication

This edition first published 2012 © 2012 by John Wiley & Sons, Inc.
First edtion © 1994 by Veterinary Learning Systems Co., Inc.

Wiley-Blackwell is an imprint of John Wiley & Sons, formed by the merger of Wiley's global Scientific, Technical and Medical business with Blackwell Publishing.

Registered office: John Wiley & Sons, Ltd, The Atrium, Southern Gate, Chichester, West Sussex, PO19 8SQ, UK

Editorial offices: 2121 State Avenue, Ames, Iowa 50014-8300, USA
The Atrium, Southern Gate, Chichester, West Sussex, PO19 8SQ, UK
9600 Garsington Road, Oxford, OX4 2DQ, UK

For details of our global editorial offices, for customer services and for information about how to apply for permission to reuse the copyright material in this book please see our website at www.wiley.com/wiley-blackwell.

Library of Congress Cataloging-in-Publication Data

Ketring, Kerry L.
   Atlas of feline ophthalmology / Kerry L. Ketring, Mary B. Glaze. – 2nd ed.
      p. ; cm.
   Includes bibliographical references and index.
   ISBN 978-0-470-95874-2 (pbk. : alk. paper)
   I. Glaze, Mary B. II. Title.
   [DNLM: 1. Eye Diseases–veterinary–Atlases.   2. Cat Diseases–Atlases. SF 986.E93]
   636.089′77–dc23

                                             2011042662

A catalogue record for this book is available from the British Library.

Wiley also publishes its books in a variety of electronic formats. Some content that appears in print may not be available in electronic books.

Set in 10/12 pt Humanist by Aptara® Inc., New Delhi, India
Printed and bound by CPI Group (UK) Ltd, Croydon, CR0 4YY

Disclaimer
The publisher and the author make no representations or warranties with respect to the accuracy or completeness of the contents of this work and specifically disclaim all warranties, including without limitation warranties of fitness for a particular purpose. No warranty may be created or extended by sales or promotional materials. The advice and strategies contained herein may not be suitable for every situation. This work is sold with the understanding that the publisher is not engaged in rendering legal, accounting, or other professional services. If professional assistance is required, the services of a competent professional person should be sought. Neither the publisher nor the author shall be liable for damages arising herefrom. The fact that an organization or Website is referred to in this work as a citation and/or a potential source of further information does not mean that the author or the publisher endorses the information the organization or Website may provide or recommendations it may make. Further, readers should be aware that Internet Websites listed in this work may have changed or disappeared between when this work was written and when it is read.

Contents

The Table of Contents is presented in outline form to make it as useful and informative as possible. The figures have been grouped into 12 main sections, each corresponding to a condition or specific area of the eye. The initial subheads identify the disease, condition, or injury. Subsequent subheads are used to define specific aspects of each figure. Some figures are referenced more than once because they depict more than one clinical sign or condition; thus the numbers of the figures do not always appear in sequential order.

Preface

Who can believe that there is no soul behind those luminous eyes!
— Théophile Gautier, French writer and critic

Has it really been 18 years since we completed our first feline atlas? Since that publication, the feline population has reached 83 million and the cat has surpassed the dog as the most popular pet in the United States. An increasing number of veterinarians cater preferentially or exclusively to feline patients. And now there is digital photography!

As before, our goal is to illustrate the normal and abnormal feline eye as seen in clinical practice. We had intended to make the first atlas timeless by concentrating on its images and excluding treatments likely to change with time. However, previously unrecognized pathogens and ongoing investigations of classical disorders have expanded the panorama of ocular disease in the cat. Approximately one-third of the 394 images in this edition are new. We have replaced a number of photos from the first edition with superior images, included more examples of common disorders, and added figures of ocular diseases that were not recognized in the feline eye in 1994. New entries include lesions of emerging systemic infections such as bartonellosis and aspergillosis and of novel agents including *Encephalitozoon cuniculi* and *Mycobacterium* spp. Examples of herpetic blepharitis and mycoplasmal keratitis suggest the familiar pathogens may be more pervasive than once supposed. Agents such as leishmania are noteworthy additions to the image bank as global travel facilitates the movement of foreign pathogens. Sclerosing pseudotumors, cystadenomas, iris abscesses, septic lens implantation, and aqueous misdirection syndrome round out the cast of recent characters impacting the feline eye.

The atlas is meant to serve as both a diagnostic reference with which to compare a patient's clinical signs and a colorful tool for educating its caregivers. Images are arranged anatomically, beginning externally with globe–orbit relationship and concluding with disorders of the retina and optic nerve. Each photo is accompanied by diagnosis, signalment, and a description of the pertinent ocular lesions. Keep in mind that some patients were examined more than 30 years ago, with clinical conclusions based on then-current differentials and testing. In light of today's expanded list of etiologies and diagnostic modalities, we concede that alternative diagnoses likely exist in some of these cases.

The table of contents outlines lesions structurally and lists each figure according to diagnosis. A new addition to the atlas is an appendix that groups figures by etiology rather than structure. This format makes it possible to retrieve every image linked to a selected agent or disease and better exposes the widespread effect of these various disorders on ocular health. As an example, lesions of lymphosarcoma can be found within the orbit, eyelid, conjunctiva, anterior uvea, retina, and optic nerve. Once a diagnosis is made (hopefully with the aid of the atlas), readers can then refer to the bibliography, available ophthalmic texts, or online resources for ever-changing therapeutic recommendations.

We are fortunate to have known these wonderful animals and their devoted families. Our thanks go to the referring veterinarians and ophthalmic colleagues who generously shared their patients, images, and expertise to help illustrate the beauty and resiliency of the feline eye. We sincerely appreciate the encouragement and support of our Wiley-Blackwell editors—Erica Judisch and Nancy Turner. We are without question indebted to Marsha Ketring, without whom this project would never have been completed. The countless hours she devoted to digitizing images archived as 2 × 2 slides and to refining colors and features to accurately recreate the original figures have made this atlas the best it can be. Frankly, her name belongs on its cover.

Kerry L. Ketring
Whitehall, Michigan

Mary Belle Glaze
Houston, Texas

Breed Predispositions to Ocular Disease

ABYSSINIAN
Progressive retinal atrophy: Rod-cone degeneration
    Narfstrom 1985; Stiles and Townsend 2007; Narfstrom et al 2009; Menotti-Raymond et al 2010

Progressive retinal atrophy: Rod-cone dysplasia
    Curtis, Barnett, Leon 1987; Stiles and Townsend 2007

BIRMAN
Corneal dermoid
    Hendy-Ibbs 1985; Stiles and Townsend 2007

BRITISH SHORTHAIR
Cataract
    Irby 1983

BURMESE
Corneal dermoid
    Hendy-Ibbs 1985; Stiles and Townsend 2007

Corneal sequestration
    Pentlarge 1989; Narfstrom 1999

Eyelid coloboma
    Koch 1979

Glaucoma
    Hampson, Smith, Bernays 2002

Lipid-laden aqueous
    Gunn-Moore, Crispin 1998

Third eyelid gland prolapse
    Chahory et al 2004; Stiles and Townsend 2007

DOMESTIC SHORTHAIR
Corneal dermoid
    Hendy-Ibbs 1985; Stiles and Townsend 2007

Lysosomal storage disease
    Stiles and Townsend 2007

HIMALAYAN
Cataract
    Rubin 1986

Corneal sequestration
    Pentlarge 1989; Morgan 1994; Narfstrom 1999

Eyelid cystadenoma
    Chaitman, van der Woerdt, Bartick 1999

KORAT
Lysosomal storage disease (GM_1 and GM_2 gangliosidosis)
    Stiles and Townsend 2007

MANX
Corneal dystrophy
    Bistner, Aguirre, Shively 1976

OCICAT
Progressive retinal atrophy: Rod-cone degeneration (*rdAc*)
    Menotti-Raymond et al 2010

PERSIAN
Chediak-Higashi syndrome (Blue smoke variety)
    Collier, Bryan, Prieur 1979

Corneal sequestration
    Pentlarge 1989; Morgan 1994; Narfstrom 1999; Featherstone and Sansom 2004

Entropion
    Narfstrom 1999; Williams and Kim 2009

Eyelid coloboma
    Bellhorn, Barnett, Henkind 1971

Eyelid cystadenoma
    Chaitman, van der Woerdt, Bartick 1999; Cantaloube, Raymond-Letron, Regnier 2004; Giudice et al 2009

Idiopathic epiphora
    Stiles and Townsend 2007

Lysosomal storage diseases
    Stiles and Townsend 2007

Progressive retinal atrophy (early onset)
    Rah et al 2005

SIAMESE
Convergent strabismus and nystagmus
    Johnson 1991

Corneal sequestration
    Pentlarge 1989; Narfstrom 1999

Glaucoma
    Jacobi, Dubielzig 2008

Lens luxation
    Olivera et al 1991

Lysosomal storage diseases
    Stiles and Townsend 2007

Periocular leukotrichia
    Scott, Miller, Griffin 2001a

Progressive retinal atrophy
    Giuliano, van der Woerdt 1999

SOMALI

Progressive retinal atrophy: Rod-cone degeneration (*rdAc*)
Narfstrom et al 2009; Menotti-Raymond et al 2010

References

Bellhorn RW, Barnett KC, Henkind P: Ocular coloboma in domestic cats. *J Am Vet Med Assoc* 159: 1015–1021, 1971.

Bistner SI, Aguirre G, Shively JN: Hereditary corneal dystrophy in the Manx cat: A preliminary report. *Invest Ophthalmol Vis Sci* 15: 15–26, 1976.

Cantaloube B, Raymond-Letron I, Regnier A: Multiple eyelid apocrine hidrocystomas in two Persian cats. *Vet Ophthalmol* 7: 121–125, 2004.

Chahory S, Crasta M, Trio S, et al: Three cases of prolapse of the nictitans gland in cats. *Vet Ophthalmol* 7: 417–419, 2004.

Chaitman J, van der Woerdt A, Bartick TE: Multiple eyelid cysts resembling apocrine hidrocystomas in three Persian and one Himalayan cat. *Vet Pathol* 36: 474–476, 1999.

Collier LL, Bryan GM, Prieur DJ: Ocular manifestations of Chediak-Higashi syndrome in four species of animals. *J Am Vet Med Assoc* 175: 587–590, 1979.

Curtis R, Barnett KC, Leon A: An early onset retinal dystrophy with dominant inheritance in the Abyssinian cat. Clinical and pathological findings. *Invest Ophthalmol Vis Sci* 28: 131–139, 1987.

Featherstone HJ, Sansom J: Feline corneal sequestra: A review of 64 cases (80 eyes) from 1993–2000. *Vet Ophthalmol* 7: 213–227, 2004.

Giudice C, Muscolo MC, Rondena M, et al: Eyelid multiple cysts of the apocrine gland of Moll in Persian cats. *J Fel Med Surg* 11: 487–491, 2009.

Giuliano EA, van der Woerdt A: Feline retinal degeneration: Clinical experience and new findings (1994–1997). *J Am Anim Hosp Assoc* 35: 511–514, 1999.

Gunn-Moore DA, Crispin SM: Unusual ocular condition in young Burmese cats. *Vet Rec* 142: 376, 1998.

Hampson ECGM, Smith RIE, Bernays ME: Primary glaucoma in Burmese cats. *Aust Vet J* 80: 672–680, 2002.

Hendy-Ibbs PM: Familial feline epibulbar dermoids. *Vet Rec* 116: 13–14, 1985.

Irby N. Hereditary cataract in the British short-hair cat. Genetics Workshop, 14th Annual Scientific Program of the Am Coll Vet Ophthalmol, Chicago IL, 1983.

Jacobi S, Dubielzig RR: Feline primary open angle glaucoma. *Vet Ophthalmol* 11: 162–165, 2008.

Johnson BW: Congenitally abnormal visual pathways of Siamese cats. *Compend Cont Educ Pract Vet* 13: 374–378, 1991.

Koch SA: Congenital ophthalmic abnormalities in the Burmese cat. *J Am Vet Med Assoc* 174: 90–91, 1979.

Menotti-Raymond M, David VA, Pflueger S, et al: Widespread retinal degenerative disease mutation (*rdAc*) discovered among a large number of popular cat breeds. *Vet J* 186: 32–38, 2010.

Morgan RV: Feline corneal sequestration: A retrospective study of 42 cases (1987–1991). *J Am Anim Hosp Assoc* 30: 24–28, 1994.

Narfstrom K: Progressive retinal atrophy in the Abyssinian cat. Clinical characteristics. *Invest Ophthalmol Vis Sci* 26: 193–200, 1985.

Narfstrom K: Hereditary and congenital ocular diseases in the cat. *J Fel Med Surg* 1: 135–141, 1999.

Narfstrom K, David V, Jarret O, et al: Retinal degeneration in the Abyssinian and Somali cat (*rdAc*): Correlation between genotype and phenotype and *rdAc* allele frequency in two continents. *Vet Ophthalmol* 12: 285–291, 2009.

Olivera DK, Riis RC, Dutton AG, et al: Feline lens displacement: A retrospective analysis of 345 cases. *Prog Vet Comp Ophthalmol* 1: 239–244, 1991.

Pentlarge VW: Corneal sequestration in cats. *Compend Contin Educ Pract Vet* 11: 24–32, 1989.

Rah H, Maggs DJ, Blankenship TN, et al: Early-onset, autosomal recessive, progressive retinal atrophy in Persian cats. *Invest Ophthalmol Vis Sci* 46: 1742–1747, 2005.

Rubin LF. Hereditary cataract in Himalayan cats. *Fel Pract* 16: 14–15, 1986.

Scott DW, Miller WH, Griffin CE: Pigmentary abnormalities, in Scott DW, Miller WH, Griffin CE (eds): *Muller & Kirk's Small Animal Dermatology*, 6th ed. St Louis, Saunders-Elsevier, 2001, pp 423–516.

Stiles J, Townsend WM: Feline ophthalmology, in Gelatt KN (ed): *Veterinary Ophthalmology*, 4th ed. Ames, IA, Blackwell Publishing, 2007, pp 1095–1164.

Williams DL, Kim J-Y: Feline entropion: A case series of 50 affected animals (2003–2008). *Vet Ophthalmol* 12: 221–226, 2009.

SECTION I
Normal Eye

Atlas of Feline Ophthalmology. Second Edition. Kerry L. Ketring and Mary Belle Glaze.
© 2012 John Wiley & Sons, Inc. Published 2012 by John Wiley & Sons, Inc.

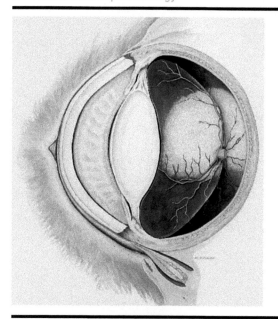

Figure 1
Cross-sectional diagram of feline eye

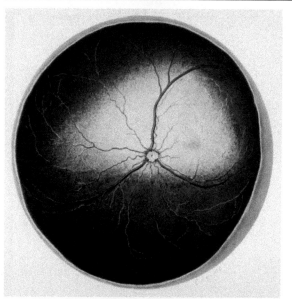

Figure 2
Fundus oculus

The entire fundus oculus of a cat's eye is represented in the artist's drawing. The nasal side is to the left and the temporal side is to the right. The brown nontapetum completely surrounds the green and yellow tapetum. The termination of the sensory retina, the ora ciliaris retinae, is represented by the pale margin surrounding the nontapetum. Peripheral to the ora is the pars plana of the ciliary body. The tapetum in the cat has a more granular appearance than in the dog. The green area in the tapetum, superior and temporal to the optic disc, represents the area centralis. The three primary venules are illustrated, two of which arch temporally. The primary venules and smaller arterioles drop off the edge of the depressed optic nerve, which is located well within the tapetum. The optic disc has a sieve-like appearance due to the structure of the lamina cribrosa.

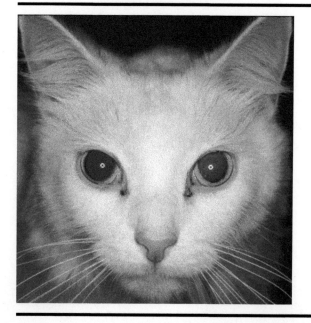

Figure 3
Heterochromia iridis
(3-year-old domestic shorthair)

In addition to the blue iris, the right eye has a red reflex through the pupil due to the atapetal fundus and lack of pigment in the retina and choroid. A typical green tapetal reflex is present in the left eye. This cat was deaf since birth, a problem linked with blue eyes and a white haircoat in domestic cats.

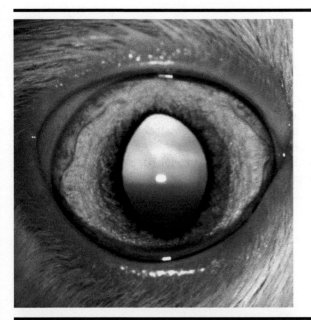

Figure 4
Normal adnexa/Anterior segment, frontal view
(1-year-old Persian)

Pictured here is the blue right eye of a white Persian, showing how little sclera is normally exposed temporally (*left side* of photograph) in the cat. Only the edge of the nictitating membrane is visible on the right. The iris vascular arcade can easily be seen against the light iris. The iris surface has a woven appearance, which is most obvious near the pupil. The pupil margin is slightly roughened because of the posterior pigmented epithelial layers, which terminate at the pupil. The red color seen through the pupil represents the reflection from the subalbinotic atapetal fundus.

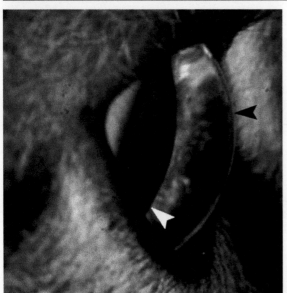

Figure 5
Normal adnexa/Anterior segment, lateral view
(3-year-old domestic shorthair)

Focused on the anterior axial cornea (*black arrow*), this photograph shows the normal corneal curvature. The anterior surface of the lens (*white arrow*) can be seen as it extends into the anterior chamber. The deep anterior chamber of the cat is the area between the arrows. Only the lateral sclera is normally visible.

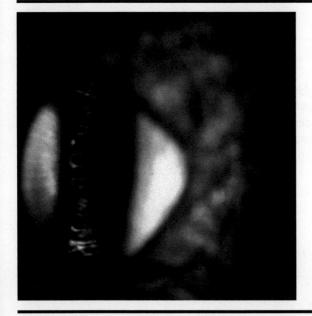

Figure 6
Normal iridocorneal angle, gross view
(2-year-old Persian)

With the camera aimed parallel to the iris face and focused at the level of the iridocorneal angle, the yellow pectinate ligaments have been brought into view. The cat's deep anterior chamber and degree of corneal curvature make it possible to see these ligaments without a gonioscopic lens.

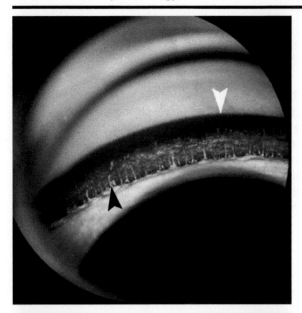

Figure 7
Normal iridocorneal angle, gonioscopic view
(3-year-old domestic shorthair)

Taken through a Koeppe goniolens, this photograph shows the normal wide drainage angle in the cat. The pectinate ligaments (*black arrow*) can be seen extending from the base of the iris to their insertion into the cornea at the termination of Descemet's membrane. The area deep to the ligaments is the trabecular meshwork. The large dark band (*white arrow*) is the superficial pigmented band representing scleral pigment.

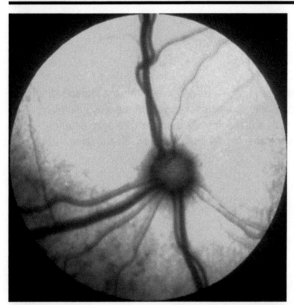

Figure 8
Normal fundus
(8-week-old domestic shorthair)

The immature tapetum is blue in all cats and gradually assumes its adult coloration by 4 months of age. The optic disc appears pinker in the kitten than in the adult cat.

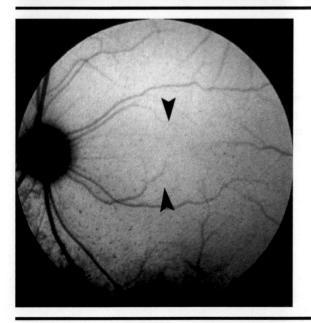

Figure 9
Normal fundus
(2-year-old domestic shorthair)

The area centralis (*arrows*) is seen temporal to the disc in this left eye. The area is cone-rich and comparatively devoid of vessels. The region is often a slightly different color than that of the surrounding tapetum, as the green color here demonstrates. The photograph was taken with a neutral density filter, causing the optic disc to appear darker than normal.

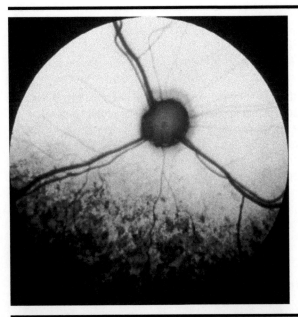

Figure 10
Normal fundus
(3-year-old Persian)

The sieve-like appearance of the optic disc is due to the lamina cribrosa. The incomplete green circle around the disc is referred to as conus and may appear hyperreflective. The normal retinal vessels, both the larger venules and the smaller arterioles, emerge near the rim of the optic disc. The cat has a complete physiologic cup at the disc's center.

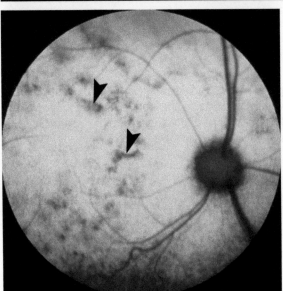

Figure 11
Normal fundus
(4-year-old Himalayan)

When the underlying choroidal pigment is exposed by thinned or hypoplastic tapetum, green and dark spots (*arrows*) are created.

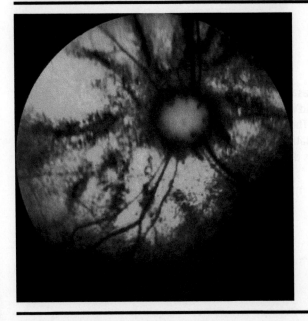

Figure 12
Normal fundus
(4-year-old domestic shorthair)

The dark red streaks seen in the tapetum are a consequence of tapetal hypoplasia. The underlying normal choroidal vessels and pigment are now more easily visualized.

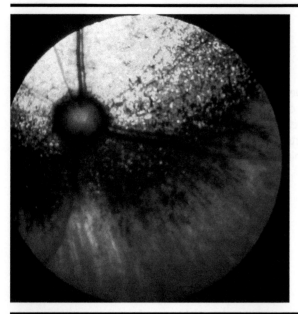

Figure 13
Normal fundus
(adult domestic shorthair)

The blue color of the immature tapetum persists in this adult cat. The inferior nontapetal area lacks pigment, allowing visualization of the normal choroidal vessels.

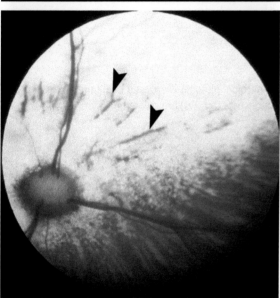

Figure 14
Normal fundus
(4-year-old Siamese)

Focal tapetal hypoplasia exposes choroidal vessels, producing red streaks and dots (*arrows*) within the tapetal fundus. Lack of pigment in the inferior nontapetal area allows the normal choroidal vessels to be seen. Both findings are normal in the Siamese and other color-dilute breeds.

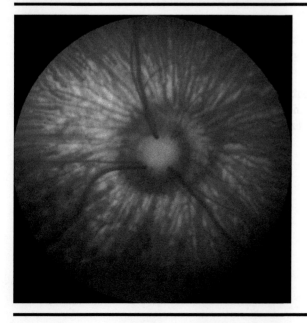

Figure 15
Normal fundus
(4-year-old domestic shorthair)

This white cat has no tapetum. Pigment in the retinal pigmented epithelium (RPE) and choroid is also sparse. With these variations, the choroidal vessels are easily seen. The shaded area surrounding the optic disc may be a subalbinotic variation of conus. Normal retinal vessels span the area but choroidal vessels decrease in density.

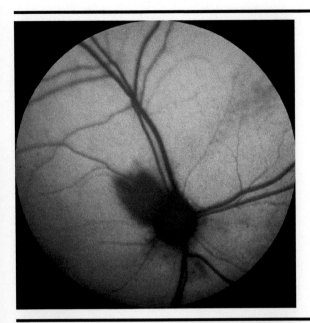

Figure 16
Normal fundus
(12-year-old domestic shorthair)

Excessive myelin radiates from the disc surface into the surrounding nerve fiber layer, creating a feathered or flame-shaped pattern distally. This was a unilateral finding in this patient, but the variation does occur bilaterally.

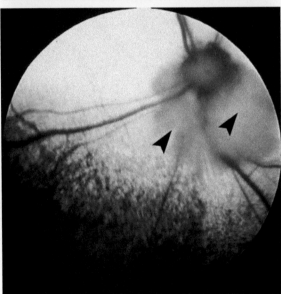

Figure 17
Normal fundus
(11-year-old domestic shorthair)

Excessive myelin anterior to the lamina cribrosa radiates from the disc in the nerve fiber layer (*arrows*). Some retinal vessels are covered by the myelin. The variation was present in both eyes of this cat.

SECTION II
Globe–Orbit Relationship

Atlas of Feline Ophthalmology. Second Edition. Kerry L. Ketring and Mary Belle Glaze.
© 2012 John Wiley & Sons, Inc. Published 2012 by John Wiley & Sons, Inc.

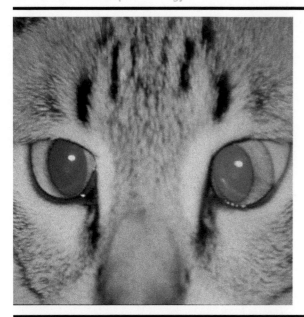

Figure 18
Convergent strabismus
(adult domestic shorthair)

The medial deviation of the globes produces a crossed-eye appearance and exposes more lateral sclera than usual. The cat has no recognizable visual deficit. The red color of the pupils is a result of limited choroidal pigmentation in this blue-eyed patient.

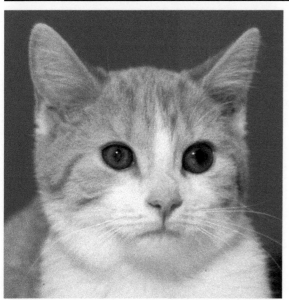

Figure 19
Microphthalmia
(6-month-old domestic shorthair)

The owners sought to explain a difference in size between the two eyes. The right eye is smaller than normal. A resorbing cataract lends a cloudy appearance to the right pupil and prevents visualization of the fundus. The left eye is normal.

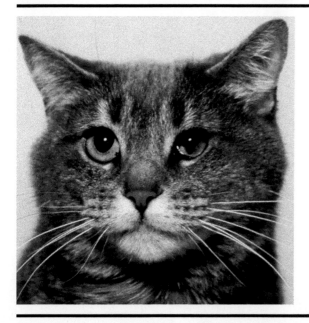

Figure 20
Phthisis bulbi
(6-year-old domestic shorthair)

Severe anterior uveitis developed in the left eye when this cat was hit by a car 3 years prior to this photograph. Ptosis of the upper lid reduces the palpebral fissure. The black margin of the third eyelid covers the medial aspect of the smaller-than-normal globe. The iris is darker and intraocular pressure is low due to prior inflammation. Multiple iris cysts were present but not visible in the photo. The pupil is irregular with no direct or indirect pupillary light reflexes (PLR). This is a blind but pain-free eye. The normal right eye also had no indirect PLR.

(Reproduced from *Veterinary Ocular Pathology: A Comparative Review*. Dubielzig, Ketring, McLellan, Albert. Elsevier Limited, 2010.)

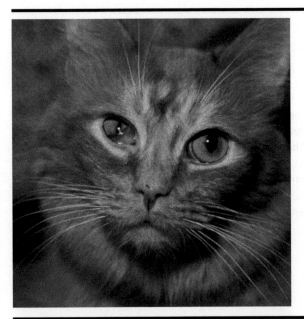

Figure 21
Horner's syndrome
(6-year-old domestic longhair)

Presented for evaluation because of a film on the right eye, this cat demonstrates an enophthalmic globe and protrusion of the nictitating membrane. Ptosis of the superior lid results in a reduced palpebral fissure. The pupil is miotic and does not dilate in dim light, despite normal direct and indirect pupillary light reflexes. The nictitans retracted following application of topical dilute phenylephrine. Thoracic radiographs suggested a mediastinal mass but owners declined further investigation.

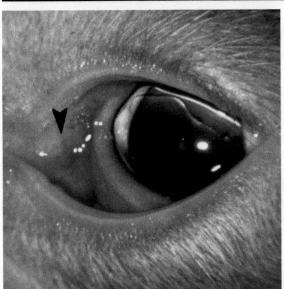

Figure 22
Prolapsed nictitans/Retrobulbar tumor
(3-year-old domestic shorthair)

The referring veterinarian treated this cat for conjunctivitis over a period of several weeks. Recently, the globe recessed and the nictitans became prominent. A firm mass (*arrow*) is palpable between the prolapsed nictitans and the orbital rim, pushing the globe posteriorly and indenting its posterior surface (see Figure 374). A needle aspirate of the mass was interpreted as a poorly differentiated sarcoma.

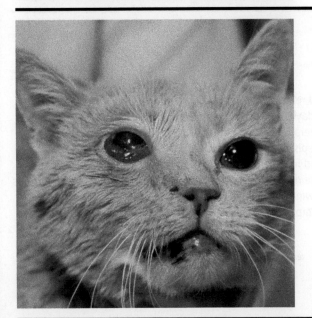

Figure 23
Retrobulbar abscess
(8-year-old domestic shorthair)

This was an outdoor cat whose owners were unaware of the duration of the condition. The conjunctiva is severely chemotic and hyperemic. The globe is exophthalmic and cannot be easily retropulsed into the orbit. Intraocular structures are normal. On oral examination, a large, swollen hemorrhagic area was found in the posterior upper dental arcade.

(Reproduced from *Veterinary Ocular Pathology: A Comparative Review*. Dubielzig, Ketring, McLellan, Albert. Elsevier Limited, 2010.)

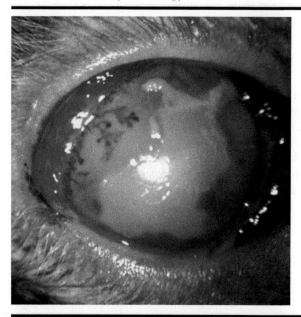

Figure 24
Retrobulbar abscess
(3-year-old Persian)

This right eye has been irritated for several weeks but recently enlarged, according to the owner. The globe is exophthalmic, painful when palpated, and difficult to retropulse. The blink response is incomplete, resulting in lagophthalmos. The conjunctiva is severely hyperemic and chemotic. The cornea has diffuse edema, a large superficial axial ulcer (stained with fluorescein dye), and vascularization. Intraocular structures were difficult to evaluate but intraocular pressure was normal. The cause of the abscess could not be determined.

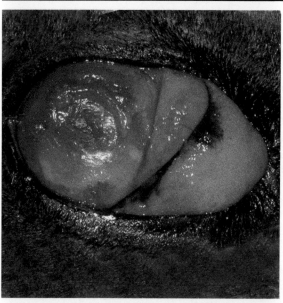

Figure 25
Orbital aspergillosis
(12-year-old Persian)

This cat was referred with a 2-month history of sneezing and bilateral nasal discharge. The biopsy-confirmed lymphoplasmacytic rhinitis resolved with oral prednisone therapy. Two months after treatment stopped, the rhinitis recurred and the right eye appeared swollen. In the photograph, the globe is exophthalmic and deviated laterally. The third eyelid protrudes, with its bulbar conjunctiva swollen beyond the nictitans' pigmented leading margin. The exposed and desiccated cornea is centrally ulcerated and discolored a light brown, with diffuse edema and intense stromal vascularization. Intraocular detail is obscured. A fine-needle aspirate of the right orbit revealed pyogranulomatous inflammation and *Aspergillus* spp hyphae.

(Image courtesy of Laura Barachetti, DVM; Barachetti L, Mortellaro CM, Giancamillo MD, Giudice C, Martino P, Travetti O, Miller PE: Bilateral orbital and nasal aspergillosis in a cat. *Vet Ophthalmol* 12(3):176–182, 2009.)

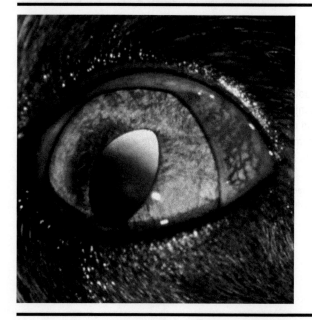

Figure 26
Retrobulbar lymphoma
(7-year-old domestic shorthair)

The owners and referring veterinarian thought this left eye had enlarged over the last 5 days. The globe is prominent, as evidenced by the amount of visible sclera laterally. The only abnormality of the anterior segment is the accompanying episcleral vascular congestion. The pupillary light responses were normal and intraocular pressure (IOP) was 26 mm Hg, interpreted as high normal. The right eye IOP measured 20 mm Hg. A retrobulbar mass was suspected following the ophthalmoscopic examination (see Figure 373) and diagnosed as lymphoma at necropsy.

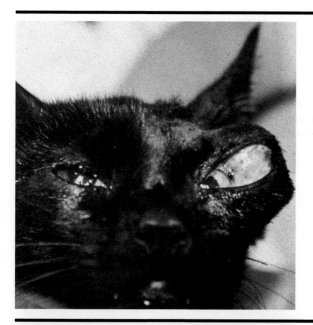

Figure 27
Zygomatic osteoma
(11-year-old domestic shorthair)

A mass lateral to the left eye had enlarged over an 8-week period, distorting the lateral canthus and preventing eyelid closure. The mass was hard, irregular, and nonpainful. Radiography confirmed a single bony mass involving the facial zygomatic bone. Excisional biopsy provided tissue for the histopathologic diagnosis of osteoma.

(Image courtesy of Robert H. Foley, DVM, DABVP; Foley RH: Zygomatic osteoma in a cat. *Feline Pract* 21:26, 1993.)

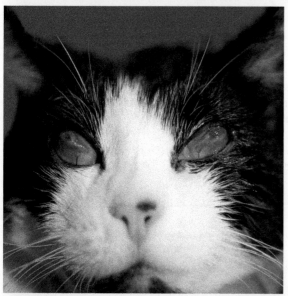

Figure 28
Orbital sclerosing pseudotumor
(12-year-old domestic shorthair)

This patient presented with a complaint of bilateral nonhealing corneal ulcers. Both globes are immobile and lid closure is incomplete. Large vessels extend from the edematous peripheral corneas toward central areas of intense vascularization. The desiccated, discolored centers of these axial lesions rise well above the surrounding tissue. The horizontal orientation mimics the shape of the palpebral fissures and suggests exposure as a factor in the chronic ulceration. The patient was euthanized 11 months later as a consequence of its unremitting orbital disease.

(Image courtesy of Marjorie H. Neaderland, DVM, DACVO.)

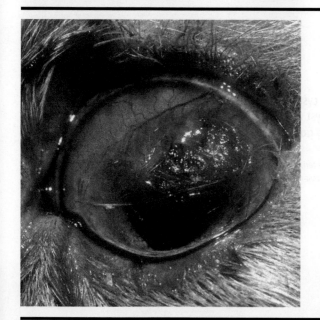

Figure 29
Orbital sclerosing pseudotumor
(adult Persian)

This patient presented with a red, cloudy left eye of unknown duration. The globe is exophthalmic and resists both forced duction and retropulsion. The eyelids are also fixed in position and unable to close over the corneal surface. Retraction of the upper lid accounts for the increased visibility of the dorsal sclera. A brownish plaque of dried exudate and desiccated tissue characterizes the exposed corneal surface. Other signs include conjunctival hyperemia, corneal edema, and superficial vascularization. Over time, the opposite eye was also affected and equally refractory to therapy.

(Image courtesy of RB Mould, BA, BVSc, CertVOphthal, MRCVS; Billson FM, Miller-Michau T, Mould JRB, Davidson MG: Idiopathic sclerosing orbital pseudotumor in seven cats. *Vet Ophthalmol* 9(1), 45–51, 2006.)

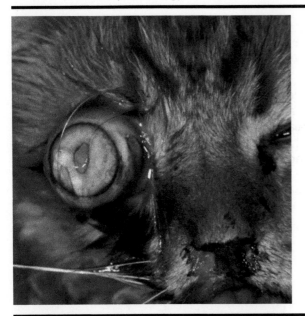

Figure 30
Traumatic proptosis
(4-year-old domestic shorthair)

Severe head trauma occurred when the cat was hit by a car. The right globe is completely displaced from the orbit and is trapped anterior to the lid margins. Multiple cranial and mandibular fractures were also identified in this patient.

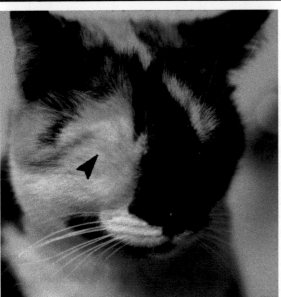

Figure 31
Orbital mucocele
(7-year-old domestic shorthair)

The right globe was enucleated due to trauma 3 months prior to this photograph. The arrow points to the area over the bony orbit where a soft swelling subsequently developed.

(Reproduced from *Veterinary Ocular Pathology: A Comparative Review*. Dubielzig, Ketring, McLellan, Albert. Elsevier Limited, 2010.)

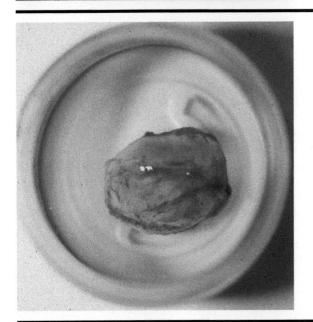

Figure 32
Orbital mucocele
(7-year-old domestic shorthair)

This thin-walled cystic structure was dissected from the orbit of the patient in Figure 31. The cyst wall was lined by conjunctival epithelium containing mucin-producing goblet cells.

(Reproduced from *Veterinary Ocular Pathology: A Comparative Review*. Dubielzig, Ketring, McLellan, Albert. Elsevier Limited, 2010.)

SECTION III

Adnexa

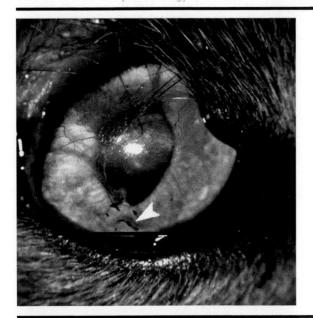

Figure 33
Eyelid agenesis/Persistent pupillary membranes (PPM)
(6-month-old domestic shorthair)

The temporal two-thirds of the superior lid margin is absent. Superficial vascularization and pigmentation are present in the superior cornea. The white arrow points to an area of endothelial pigmentation attributed to PPMs.

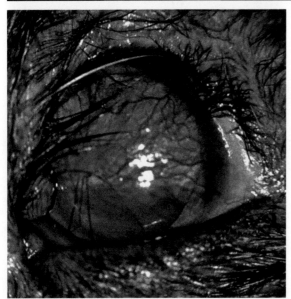

Figure 34
Eyelid agenesis
(6-month-old domestic shorthair)

Almost the entire upper lid margin is absent. Misdirected facial hairs can be seen in contact with the corneal surface. Severe corneal vascularization is evident against the tapetal reflection, a consequence of both trichiasis and exposure.

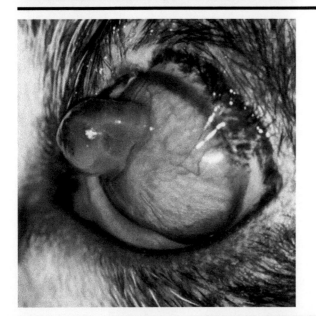

Figure 35
Eyelid agenesis/Iris prolapse
(5-month-old domestic shorthair)

The lateral two-thirds of the superior lid margin failed to develop and the cornea ulcerated due to exposure and irritation by misdirected hairs. Pigmented iris is seen extending above the corneal surface through a ruptured descemetocele. Superficial corneal vessels are highlighted against the yellow iris. The anterior chamber is flat, with the iris in close proximity to the inner cornea. The pupil is not visible.

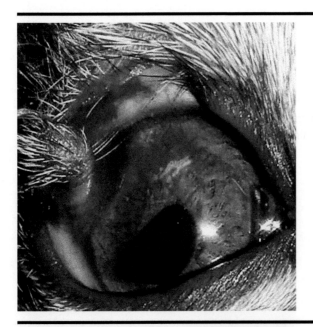

Figure 36
Eyelid agenesis/Dermoid/Iris coloboma
(3-month-old domestic shorthair)

Multiple congenital ocular anomalies are present in this kitten. The temporal half of the upper lid margin is absent and facial hairs are misdirected against the eye. A dermoid spans the lateral limbus, creating a mild opacity at its attachment to the cornea. The pupil is eccentric and misshapen owing to its colobomatous defect.

(Image courtesy of José Luiz Laus, DVM, MSc, PhD.)

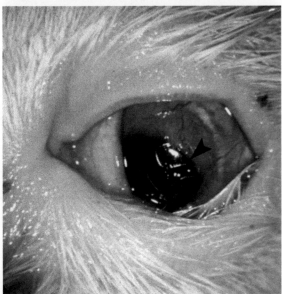

Figure 37
Entropion
(19-year-old Persian)

This cat had a lifelong history of ocular irritation and discharge. The lower eyelid is inverted, resulting in contact of the cornea by the facial hair. Prominence of the third eyelid suggests a painful eye. Superficial corneal vascularization accompanies a darkly colored sequestrum (*arrow*) in the central cornea.

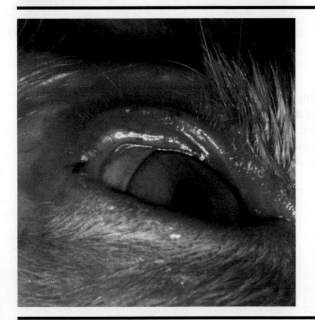

Figure 38
Cicatricial ectropion
(9-month-old domestic shorthair)

When rescued from an industrial site as a kitten, this patient's haircoat was plastered with a thick black substance resembling crude oil and the skin beneath was ulcerated. Copious mucopurulent discharge, severe conjunctivitis, and extensive superficial corneal ulceration were present bilaterally. The ocular sequelae of the chemical injury can be seen months later, with alopecia and thinning of the periocular skin. Tissue contracture compromises lid function and creates a secondary ectropion, with eversion of the upper lid margin and palpebral conjunctiva. Corneal scarring and superficial vascularization are also present, consequences of both the initial ulceration and current lagophthalmos.

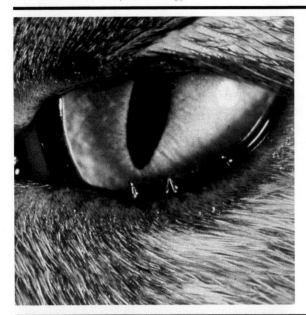

Figure 39
Distichiasis
(adult domestic shorthair)

A slight serous discharge from the left eye was a recurring complaint. Several cilia extend from the meibomian gland openings along the lower eyelid margin. The remainder of the ocular examination was unremarkable.

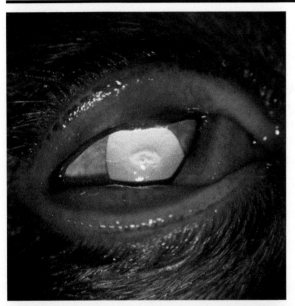

Figure 40
Herpetic blepharitis
(1-year-old domestic shorthair)

This patient was adopted from a municipal shelter at approximately 12 weeks of age, with bilateral ocular discharge and occasional sneezing that resolved within a week. From time to time, a mild discharge had been noted from the right eye. One week prior to presentation, that same eye appeared acutely painful, red, and swollen. The eyelid margins are erythematous and thickened, and marginal pigmentation is decreased. The palpebral conjunctiva is hyperemic and chemotic. Third eyelid prominence attests to the cat's discomfort. A corneal ulcer is present centrally, highlighted by the tapetal reflection. Clinical signs improved quickly with antiviral therapy.

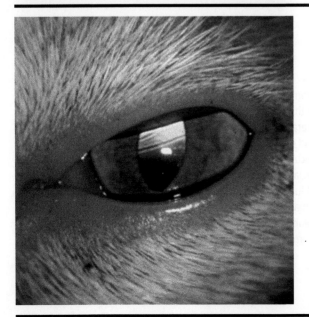

Figure 41
Allergic blepharitis
(4-month-old domestic shorthair)

The owners of this cat observed increasing discomfort and redness of the eyelids following the use of a topical tetracycline ointment prescribed for mild conjunctivitis. The cat is squinting and the lid margins are hyperemic. Edematous conjunctiva can be seen extending beyond the superior lid margin. All signs resolved when topical medication was discontinued.

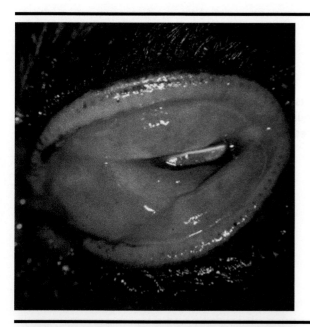

Figure 42
Allergic blepharitis/Conjunctivitis
(2-year-old domestic shorthair)

In spite of progressively worsening blepharospasm, the owner continued to apply trifluridine several times daily to treat a herpetic ulcer. As a consequence, the lid margins are inflamed and depigmented. Severe conjunctival hyperemia and chemosis combine with the prominent third eyelid to obscure the cornea.

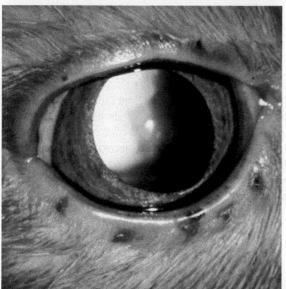

Figure 43
Bacterial blepharitis
(5-year-old domestic shorthair)

Both lids of each eye were focally hyperemic with punctate abscesses below the lid margins. *Staphylococcus* spp was cultured from the lesions.

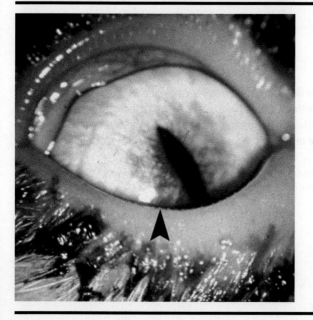

Figure 44
Meibomianitis
(6-month-old Persian)

The lid margins appear roughened due to the presence of fine caseous plugs (*arrow*) at the openings of the meibomian glands. Copious dark periocular discharge, conjunctival hyperemia, and chemosis accompany the lid changes. Swabs of meibomian secretions and the conjunctival surface failed to identify any bacterial, viral, or fungal etiology.

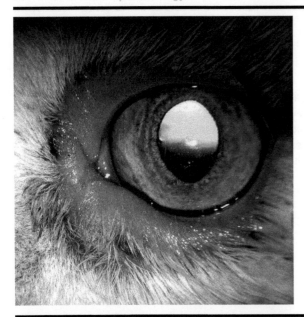

Figure 45
Apocrine cystadenoma/Hidrocystoma
(1-year-old Persian)

This patient exhibits only mildly elevated gray to black lesions near the lower lid margin and medial canthus, typical of the early stages of this disorder. Lesions were present bilaterally.

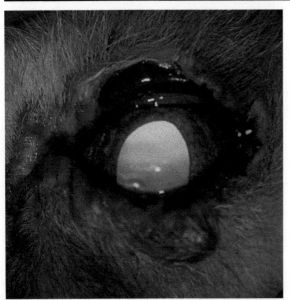

Figure 46
Apocrine cystadenoma/Hidrocystoma
(10-year-old Persian)

The owner first noted a small, dark gray swelling near the medial canthus of the left eye 8 months prior to presentation. Over time variable-sized nodules developed within the eyelids of both eyes. No other dermatologic lesions were present. Multiple dark gray to black soft, fluid-filled cysts are present in the upper and lower eyelids of the more severely affected left eye. Fine-needle aspiration of a larger lesion collapsed the swelling, producing a small quantity of brown fluid containing red blood cells, nondegenerate neutrophils, and macrophages.

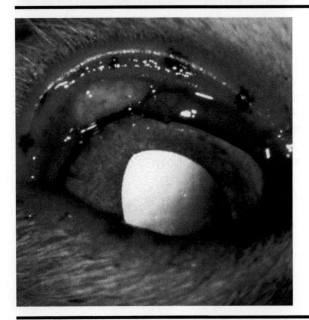

Figure 47
Chalazion
(5-year-old domestic shorthair)

A large white swelling beneath the superior palpebral conjunctiva can be seen in this cat with chronic conjunctivitis. A firm caseous material compatible with that of inspissated meibomian gland secretions was curetted from the mass.

(Reproduced from *Veterinary Ocular Pathology: A Comparative Review*. Dubielzig, Ketring, McLellan, Albert. Elsevier Limited, 2010.)

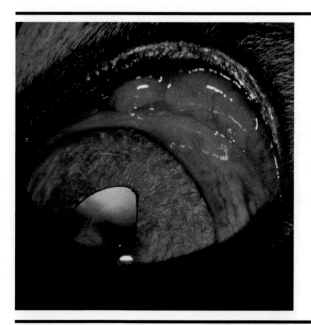

Figure 48
Lipogranulomatous conjunctivitis
(12-year-old domestic shorthair)

This bilateral disease was restricted to the inner surface of the upper eyelids. The palpebral conjunctiva is mildly hyperemic and distended in subtly lobulated fashion. Multiple distinct white nodules were present in the contralateral eye, a classical feature attributed to accumulations of lipid-laden macrophages or leaking meibomian secretions beneath the conjunctiva.

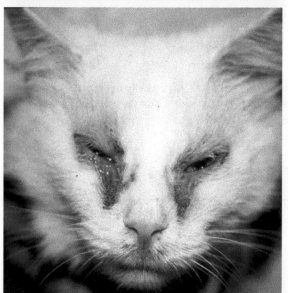

Figure 49
Demodicosis
(13-year-old domestic longhair)

Blepharitis in this diabetic cat is characterized by exudative dermatitis, alopecia, erosion, and crusting. The eyes were normal. Periocular skin scrapings were positive for *Demodex* spp.

(Image courtesy of Barbara A. Kummel, DVM.)

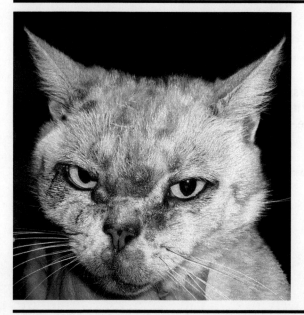

Figure 50
Mycobacterial dermatitis/Blepharitis
(5-year-old domestic longhair)

This indoor/outdoor cat was known by the owners as an aggressive hunter. Multiple pink to gray nodules can be seen on the face, a few of which are encroaching within the medial canthus of the right eye. Similar lesions were also present on the paws. The nodules were located in the subcutis and were not painful, hot, or ulcerated. The granulomas were caused by *Mycobacterium* sp. strain *Tarwin*.

(Image courtesy of Janet A. Fyfe, BSc (Hons), PhD; Fyfe JA, McCowan C, O'Brien CR, et al: Molecular characterization of a novel fastidious mycobacterium causing lepromatous lesions of the skin, subcutis, cornea, and conjunctiva of cats living in Victoria, Australia. *Clin Microbiol* 46(2):618–626, 2007.)

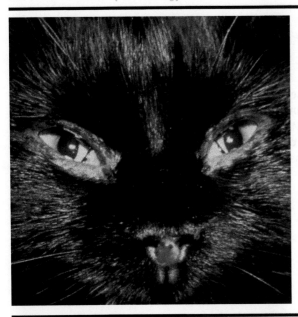

Figure 51
Allergic blepharitis
(2-year-old domestic shorthair)

The owners observed irritation around the eyes and nose 3 days after starting tetracycline/polymyxin B (Terramycin®) ophthalmic ointment, but continued treatment for a total of 7 days, when this photograph was taken. The lids and nasal planum are hyperemic and ulcerated. All lesions significantly improved 3 days after discontinuing the topical medication.

(Image courtesy of David T. Ramsey, DVM, MS, DACVO.)

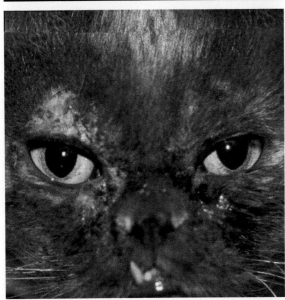

Figure 52
Food allergy
(4-year-old Persian)

Pruritus and constant rubbing led to this cat's patchy periocular alopecia and excoriation. Exudative facial fold dermatitis is also present. Food allergy was suspected on the basis of clinical signs and confirmed by a food elimination trial.

(Image courtesy of Barbara A. Kummel, DVM.)

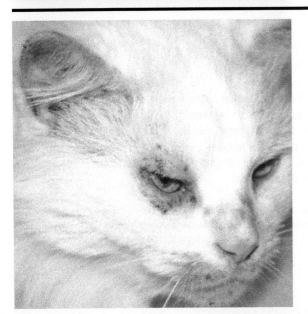

Figure 53
Pemphigus erythematosus
(adult domestic longhair)

The left eyelids are spared the erythematous macular dermatitis and excoriations of the right periocular region. Combined with those of the nose, muzzle, and pinnae, these periocular lesions are compatible with pemphigus erythematosus.

(Image courtesy of Barbara A. Kummel, DVM.)

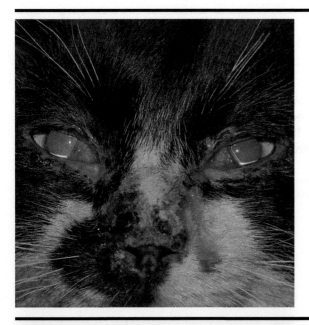

Figure 54
Herpetic blepharitis/Dermatitis
(2-year-old American shorthair)

This cat was adopted from a shelter at 8 weeks of age. Lymphadenopathy and fever of unknown origin developed 4 months prior to presentation. Following a thorough diagnostic workup to rule out infectious disease, systemic corticosteroid therapy was begun. The fever resolved with treatment but daily therapy was required to prevent relapses. Three weeks after beginning steroids, ocular discharge and redness developed. A bacterial infection was diagnosed based on culture but ocular signs persisted despite antibiotic therapy. Accompanying nasal lesions were incorrectly attributed to the constant ocular discharge. At examination, both eyes are painful, with squinting and third eyelid protrusion. The eyelids are erythematous, with alopecia, marginal erosions, and crusting. Similar lesions extend to the nasal planum. Dendritic corneal lesions were present bilaterally but are not visible in the photo. The ocular and skin lesions improved rapidly with antiviral therapy.

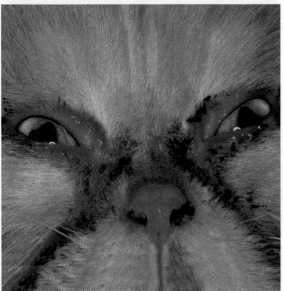

Figure 55
Idiopathic facial dermatitis of Persians
(4-year-old Persian)

This cat had a long history of black ocular discharge that required daily cleansing. Increasing redness of the eyelids and facial folds began 1 year ago. Yeast and cocci were identified cytologically but antimicrobial therapy failed to resolve the problem. Lesions surrounding the eyes and along the facial folds are characterized by black exudates adherent to the skin and hair, with erythema and excoriation of the underlying skin. This incurable dermatologic disorder has been misinterpreted as facial scalding related to excessive ocular discharge.

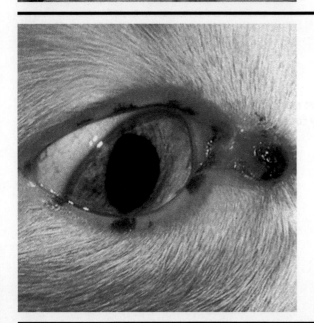

Figure 56
Cutaneous histiocytosis
(11-year-old domestic longhair)

The owners noticed this medial canthal mass for about 1 month. The raised, firm, nonpigmented, and ulcerated mass measures approximately 5 × 7 mm. There was no conjunctival involvement. Histopathology diagnosed a progressive dendritic cell histiocytosis.

(Image courtesy of Paige M. Evans, DVM.)

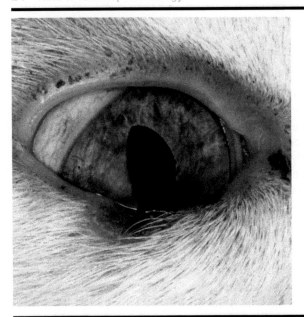

Figure 57
Squamous cell carcinoma
(12-year-old domestic shorthair)

According to the owner, this red spot on the lower eyelid gradually enlarged over a 3-month period. The lid margin is notched by an erythematous, ulcerative lesion. The right eyelid, nasal planum, and pinnae of both ears were similarly affected.

(Reproduced from *Veterinary Ocular Pathology: A Comparative Review*. Dubielzig, Ketring, McLellan, Albert. Elsevier Limited, 2010.)

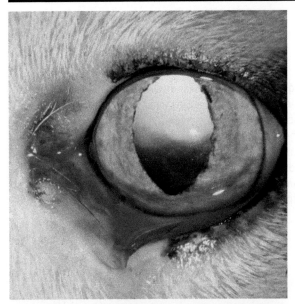

Figure 58
Squamous cell carcinoma
(12-year-old domestic shorthair)

The medial canthus and nasal one-third of the lower lid are eroded by the tumor. The bulbar conjunctiva is normal. Biopsy confirmed the diagnosis.

(Reproduced from *Veterinary Ocular Pathology: A Comparative Review*. Dubielzig, Ketring, McLellan, Albert. Elsevier Limited, 2010.)

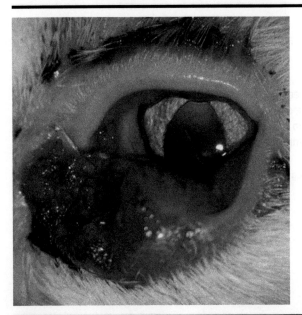

Figure 59
Squamous cell carcinoma
(17-year-old domestic shorthair)

This large erosive mass involved the lower lid, palpebral conjunctiva and nictitans. Biopsy confirmed the diagnosis.

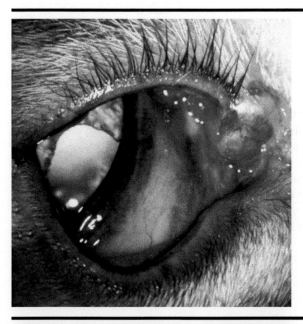

Figure 60
Adenocarcinoma
(16-year-old Abyssinian)

A firm, irregularly lobulated mass distorts the superior nasal lid and palpebral conjunctiva. The nictitating membrane was spared. Biopsy confirmed the diagnosis.

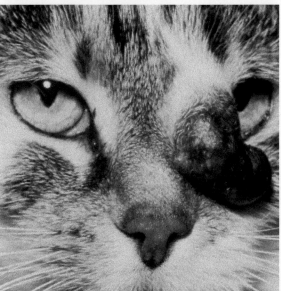

Figure 61
Adenocarcinoma
(14-year-old domestic shorthair)

A slow-growing mass had been observed for 5 years by the owners of this cat. The elongate mass resembles a proboscis, attached at its base near the medial canthus but free of surrounding tissue at its distal (inferior) end. The eyelid margin near the medial canthus was spared. Histopathology confirmed the diagnosis.

(Image courtesy of Denise Lindley, DVM, MS, DACVO.)

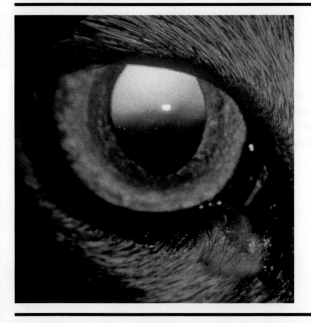

Figure 62
Mast cell tumor
(7-year-old domestic shorthair)

Four months ago, the owner noted a pink swelling near this cat's medial canthus. The lesion remained unchanged until a crust developed on its surface a few days prior to presentation. The pink, relatively hairless mass is raised above the surrounding tissue. An area of ulceration along its upper margin is deeper red in color. Fine-needle aspiration revealed a homogeneous population of mast cells.

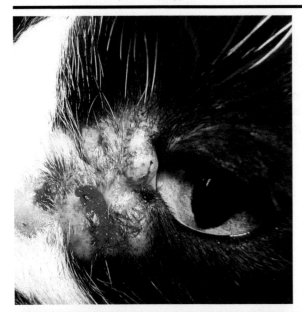

Figure 63
Mast cell tumor
(9-year-old domestic shorthair)

This lesion increased in size over a period of 9 months. A pink, firm, multilobulated, alopecic, and ulcerated mass encircles the medial canthus and extends onto the bridge of the nose. Diagnosis was based on cytology of a fine-needle aspirate and later confirmed histopathologically. Preoperative blood work and thoracic radiography were normal. No recurrence was seen in the 6 months following surgery that combined enucleation, tumor resection, and skin grafting.

(Image courtesy of Jean Stiles, DVM, MS, DACVO.)

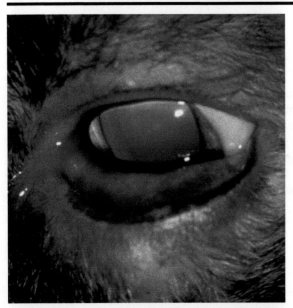

Figure 64
Mast cell tumor
(8-year-old Siamese)

The entire lower lid was distorted by soft swelling. The inferior palpebral conjunctiva is hyperemic and elevated by the tumor. Cytologic evaluation of a fine-needle aspirate confirmed the diagnosis.

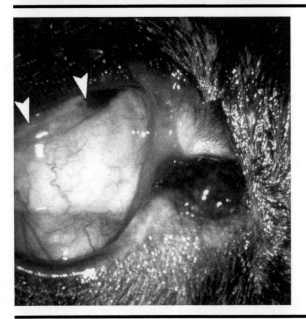

Figure 65
Melanoma
(10-year-old Siamese)

This black mass had been present for an unspecified period of time. It is well delineated from surrounding tissue within the medial canthus. The third eyelid (*arrows*) has been intentionally prolapsed for the photograph. Melanoma was diagnosed following histopathology of the surgically excised tissue.

(Image courtesy of Art J. Quinn, DVM, DACVO.)

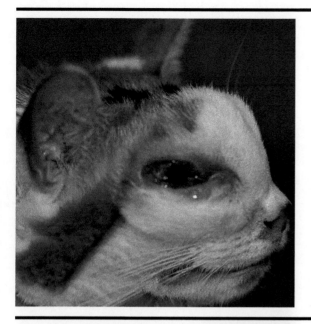

Figure 66
Periorbital lymphoma
(9-year-old domestic shorthair)

Facial swelling had been present for 2 months, but this cat appeared otherwise healthy prior to presentation. The swelling is reasonably circumscribed, surrounding the right eye and extending across the bridge of the nose. The eyelid margins and conjunctiva are hyperemic but the globe itself is unaffected despite reduced lid mobility. A fine-needle aspirate of the subcutaneous tissue confirmed the diagnosis of lymphoma. No other lesions of lymphoma were identified.

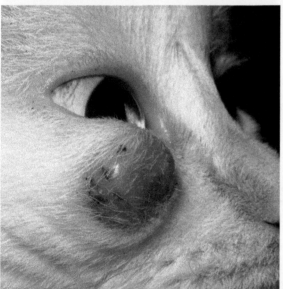

Figure 67
Peripheral nerve sheath tumor
(middle-aged adult domestic shorthair)

Local shelter personnel had no history regarding this patient or its periocular swelling. A large subcutaneous tumor distorts the lower lid. The overlying skin appears thin and hairless. Physical examination was otherwise unremarkable. The tumor type was determined on biopsy. Additional staging and treatment were declined.

(Image courtesy of Jean Stiles, DVM, MS, DACVO.)

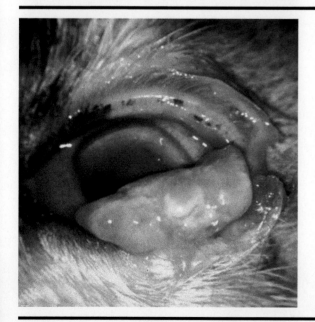

Figure 68
Granuloma/Histoplasmosis
(8-year-old domestic shorthair)

Mucopurulent discharge accompanies a proliferative, hyperemic lesion along the lower eyelid. The bulbar and third eyelid conjunctiva are also hyperemic, but intraocular detail is difficult to visualize. *Histoplasma* organisms were identified in this granulomatous lid lesion. Anterior uveitis and chorioretinitis (see Figures 204 and 312) were also present, along with oral and cutaneous lesions.

SECTION IV
Conjunctiva

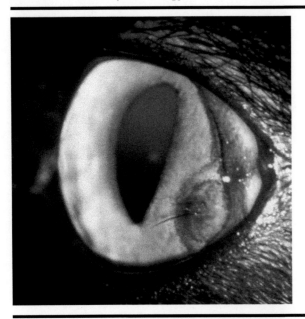

Figure 69
Dermoid
(3-year-old Burmese)

An abnormally located patch of skin extends onto the cornea from the temporal limbus. Several cilia arise from follicles within the lightly pigmented surface. This is both a congenital and inherited disease in this breed.

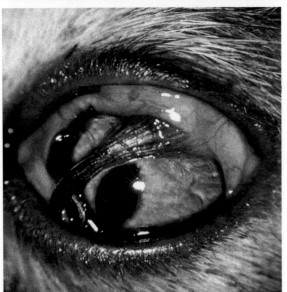

Figure 70
Dermoid
(13-week-old Persian)

Increased tearing called attention to this eye with a dermoid in an unusual dorsal location. Long hairs extend across the central cornea, originating from hair follicles based solely within the bulbar conjunctiva. The deeper sclera and cornea were unaffected.

(Reproduced from *Veterinary Ocular Pathology: A Comparative Review*. Dubielzig, Ketring, McLellan, Albert. Elsevier Limited, 2010.)

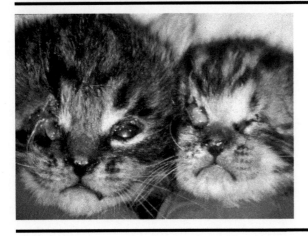

Figure 71
Neonatal ophthalmia
(2.5-week-old domestic shorthair)

Only these two kittens survived of a litter of six. Their poor general health was blamed on an upper respiratory infection complicated by malnutrition. In the smaller kitten, exudate is trapped beneath the closed lids, with secondary swelling. Purulent material seeps through the partially opened palpebral fissure of the right eye. The larger kitten's open eye is superficially ulcerated and vascularized, though lesions are not apparent in the photo. The right eye is obscured by exudate. Feline herpesvirus and secondary bacterial opportunists were the presumed pathogens.

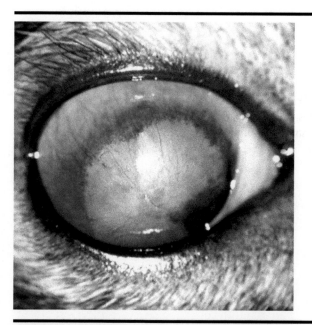

Figure 72
Symblepharon
(8-year-old domestic shorthair)

Rescued as a kitten with severe upper respiratory disease, this patient's cloudy right eye had remained unchanged through the years. Conjunctival vessels cross the unusually pigmented limbal region and extend circumferentially onto the corneal surface. Superficial pigment further obscures the iris near the prominent third eyelid. The symblepharon-related corneal pigmentation and vascularization are indicative of the prior herpetic infection.

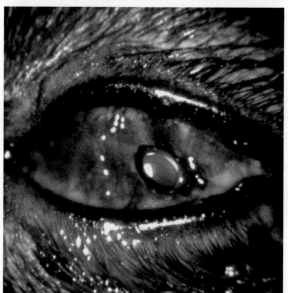

Figure 73
Symblepharon
(11-month-old domestic shorthair)

At 2 months of age, this patient was treated for bilateral herpetic keratoconjunctivitis that had been present since birth. Severe adhesions of the conjunctiva extend 360 degrees, totally obscuring the third eyelid and all but the axial cornea. The blue–green tapetal reflection is seen through a small hole at the center of the adhesions.

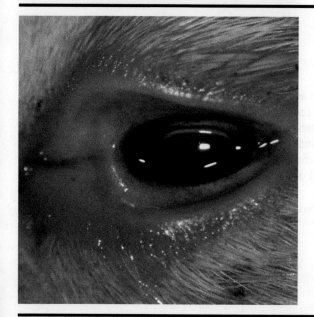

Figure 74
Median canthal symblepharon/Ankyloblepharon
(6-month-old domestic shorthair)

This patient was one of several feral kittens with upper respiratory disease rescued by an animal protection group. The respiratory signs resolved with supportive care. The left eye of this cat has since appeared smaller than normal, with constant tearing. There is extensive symblepharon formation spanning the medial canthus and palpebral fissure, reducing the length of the palpebral fissure and obliterating the nasolacrimal puncta. Palpebral conjunctiva is easily visualized along the remaining length of the lid where additional adhesions limit the depth of the conjunctival cul-de-sac. Intraocular structures were normal and the eye remained sighted.

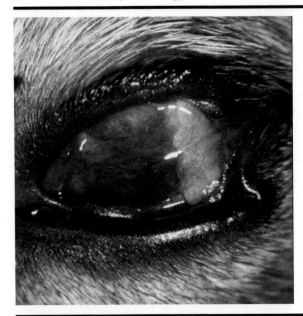

Figure 75
Symblepharon
(8-week-old Somali)

The entire litter of kittens was affected with feline herpetic keratoconjunctivitis. The conjunctival overgrowth extends from the upper and lower cul-de-sacs to cover the entire cornea and nictitans. The globe is functionally blind.

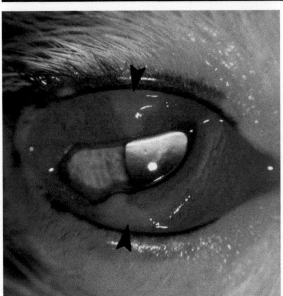

Figure 76
Herpetic conjunctivitis
(6-month-old domestic shorthair)

Similar clinical signs were present bilaterally in this young cat. The conjunctiva is severely hyperemic, with milder chemosis. The prominent third eyelid also reflects these changes and suggests the eye is painful. The arrows point to two fluorescein-positive areas on the conjunctiva that represent epithelial erosions caused by FHV-1. Lesions such as these are a factor in symblepharon formation. Neither cornea was ulcerated.

(Reproduced from *Veterinary Ocular Pathology: A Comparative Review*. Dubielzig, Ketring, McLellan, Albert. Elsevier Limited, 2010.)

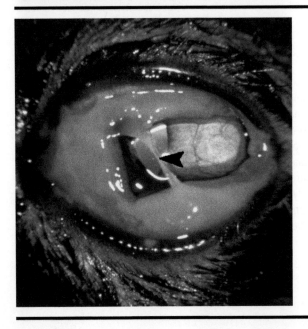

Figure 77
Herpetic conjunctivitis
(8-week-old domestic shorthair)

This kitten had an active upper respiratory infection accompanied by bilateral ocular signs. The conjunctiva is hyperemic and severely chemotic. A thick, white pseudomembrane has formed across the visible conjunctiva. A membranous strand (*arrow*) extends from the superior to inferior palpebral conjunctiva. The conjunctival surface beneath the membrane is raw, increasing the risk of permanent symblepharon.

(Reproduced from *Veterinary Ocular Pathology: A Comparative Review*. Dubielzig, Ketring, McLellan, Albert. Elsevier Limited, 2010.)

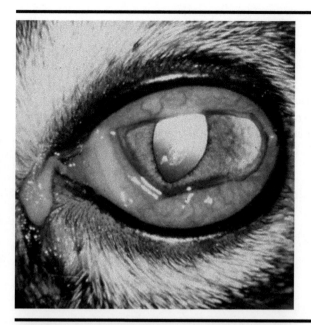

Figure 78
Chlamydophila conjunctivitis
(1-year-old domestic shorthair)

A history of periodic sneezing was associated with this bilateral condition. The conjunctiva is moderately hyperemic and chemotic. A mucopurulent discharge is present in the medial canthus. The cornea is normal. The axial opacity represents a nuclear cataract.

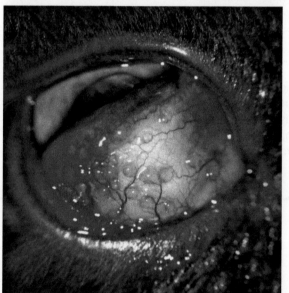

Figure 79
Chlamydophila conjunctivitis
(2-year-old Persian)

No signs of respiratory disease were seen in this patient with bilateral conjunctivitis. The third eyelid has been intentionally prolapsed to show the hyperemia and multiple lymphoid follicles found throughout the conjunctiva. An indirect fluorescent antibody test was positive for *Chlamydophila felis*.

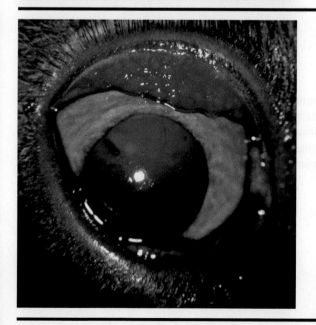

Figure 80
Chlamydophila conjunctivitis
(6-month-old Persian)

This kitten has a mild upper respiratory infection and bilateral conjunctivitis. Follicles are especially prominent within the hyperemic dorsal palpebral conjunctiva. Ocular and respiratory signs resolved with oral doxycycline therapy.

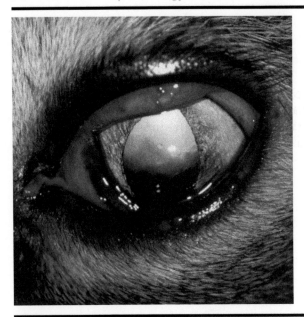

Figure 81
Bartonella conjunctivitis
(4-year-old domestic shorthair)

A mild mucoid discharge accompanies the bilateral conjunctivitis in this patient. Moderate conjunctival hyperemia and mild chemosis are seen, along with third eyelid prominence. Conjunctival scrapings submitted for PCR were negative for FHV-1, *Chlamydophila*, and *Mycoplasma*. *Bartonella* serology was positive.

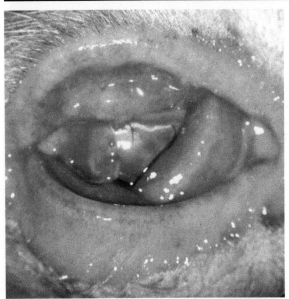

Figure 82
Mycoplasma
(8-year-old domestic shorthair)

This patient's chronic bilateral conjunctivitis is characterized by diffusely thickened and hyperemic conjunctiva and a prominent third eyelid. Moderate mucoid discharge is present along the lid margins and across the corneal surface. Conjunctival PCR was positive for *Mycoplasma* spp. PCR for FHV-1 and *Chlamydophila felis* was negative, as was serology for *Bartonella*.

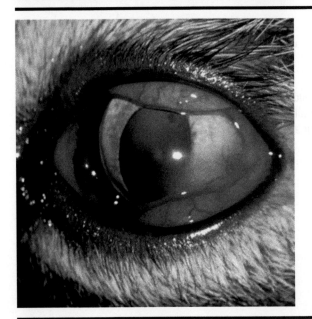

Figure 83
Herpesvirus/*Mycoplasma*/*Bartonella* conjunctivitis
(2-year-old domestic shorthair)

This patient presented with a complaint of bilateral conjunctivitis. The conjunctiva is hyperemia and chemotic, with a serous ocular discharge. In this left eye, the temporal cornea is ulcerated, edematous, and superficially vascularized. A conjunctival scraping submitted for PCR was positive for both FHV-1 and *Mycoplasma*. Serology was also positive for *Bartonella*.

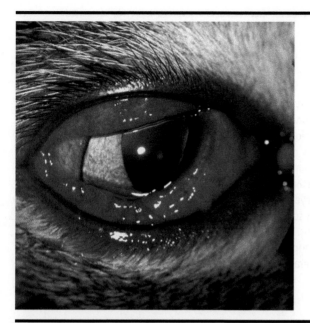

Figure 84
Chlamydophila/Bartonella conjunctivitis
(2-year-old domestic shorthair)

Intense conjunctival hyperemia and mild chemosis characterize the bilateral conjunctivitis in this patient. Slight mucoid discharge is evident overlying the prominent third eyelid. There is no active corneal disease. PCR testing on a conjunctival sample was positive for *Chlamydophila* and negative for FHV-1 and *Mycoplasma*. Serology was positive for *Bartonella*.

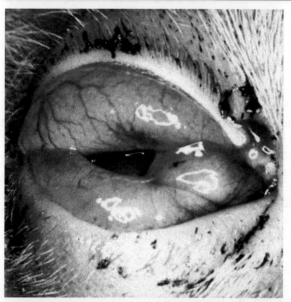

Figure 85
Allergic conjunctivitis/Insect sting
(2-year-old domestic shorthair)

The owner noted acute swelling of the periocular area shortly after seeing his cat wandering through the garden. The eye had been normal 1 hour earlier. Chemosis is the predominant feature. A small area of subconjunctival hemorrhage is present beneath the superior lid. Prominence of the nictitans is also attributed to the conjunctival edema. The globe was difficult to evaluate in its entirety but was ultimately determined to be normal as the chemosis resolved over a 24-hour period. The cause was presumed to be an insect sting, although reaction to garden chemicals could not be excluded.

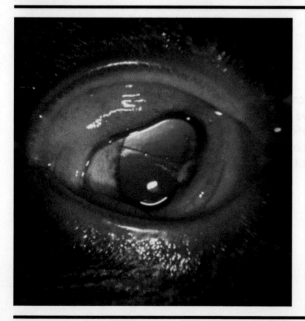

Figure 86
Eosinophilic conjunctivitis
(2-year-old Siamese)

This bilateral condition was restricted to the conjunctiva and nictitating membrane. All conjunctival surfaces are hyperemic and chemotic with a diffuse grainy appearance. Bacterial cultures and fluorescent antibody tests for feline herpesvirus and *Chlamydophila* were negative. Cytology of a conjunctival scraping revealed epithelial cells, lymphocytes, and eosinophils.

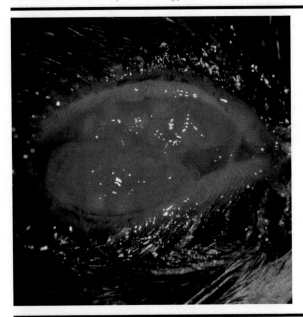

Figure 87
Eosinophilic conjunctivitis
(4-year-old domestic shorthair)

Early ocular history was unknown in this adopted patient. Intermittent episodes of conjunctivitis and ocular discharge had occurred in the right eye over a 2-year period, but clinical signs had escalated in recent weeks. Topical antibiotic therapy considered beneficial in previous episodes was no longer effective. Large lymphoid follicles create a nodular appearance to the exposed conjunctiva. In addition to marked conjunctival hyperemia and thickening, the eyelid margins are erythematous and depigmented. Cytology of a conjunctival scraping revealed eosinophils, lymphocytes, plasma cells, and macrophages. Although the eye itself could not be visualized at this initial visit, eosinophilic keratitis was evident as the conjunctival disease responded to therapy. The opposite eye was normal.

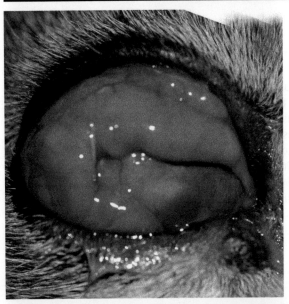

Figure 88
Leishmaniasis
(21-year-old European shorthair)

Masses affecting the eyes and mouth gradually enlarged and vision diminished in the 5 months preceding this patient's examination. Exophthalmos is accompanied by dramatic tissue proliferation that spans the limbus, creating a hyperemic, irregularly thickened mass that encircles most of the anterior globe. The adjacent cornea is infiltrated by the same flesh-colored tissue, with accompanying edema. Ocular ultrasound revealed bilateral exudative retinal detachments and extraocular myositis. Systemic signs included mild-generalized lymphadenopathy, ulcerative facial dermatitis, facial deformity, and oral mucosal masses. Leishmania amastigotes were found in a conjunctival biopsy. ELISA and RT-PCR for *Leishmania* spp were highly positive. Proliferative tissue decreased substantially following 2 months of therapy.

(Image courtesy of Teresa Pena, DVM, PhD.)

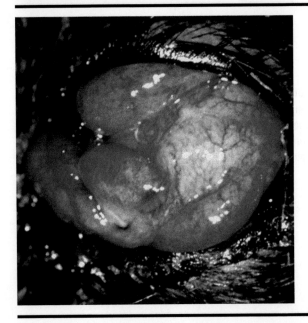

Figure 89
Blastomycosis
(6-year-old domestic shorthair)

This patient presented with a complaint of severe unilateral conjunctivitis. The cat's right eye and general health were considered within limits of normal. All conjunctival surfaces are extremely hyperemic and chemotic, making it impossible to visualize the cornea and intraocular structures. Blastomycosis was diagnosed based on histopathology of the globe.

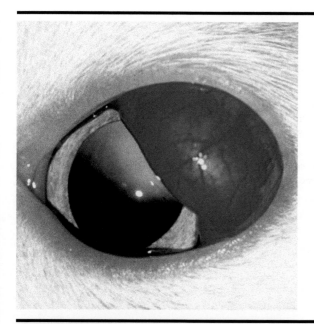

Figure 90
Histoplasmosis
(1.5-year-old domestic shorthair)

This cat was presented with progressive conjunctival swelling. A large and notably hyperemic bulbar subconjunctival mass obscures the adjacent limbus. This lesion was accompanied by a severe chorioretinitis in the opposite eye (see Figure 313). A fine-needle aspirate and biopsy of the mass identified *Histoplasma* organisms within macrophages.

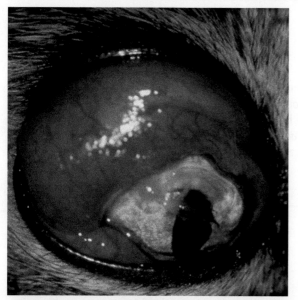

Figure 91
Lymphoma
(5-year-old Persian)

A large subconjunctival mass affecting the superior palpebral and bulbar tissues had been present for 2 weeks. Lagophthalmos resulted in exposure and secondary corneal ulceration. A smaller mass had been noted in the left eye 4 days prior to this photograph. Biopsies of both masses were consistent with lymphoma.

(Reproduced from *Veterinary Ocular Pathology: A Comparative Review*. Dubielzig, Ketring, McLellan, Albert. Elsevier Limited, 2010.)

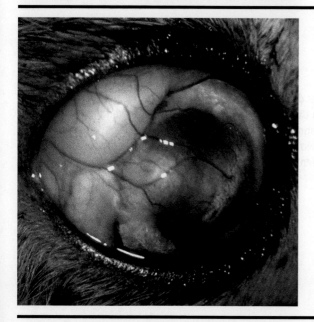

Figure 92
Conjunctival cyst
(5-year-old Persian)

This cat's ocular history was unknown. A subconjunctival mass overlies the dorsotemporal sclera. Several conjunctival vessels extend across its surface and onto an adjacent corneal opacity. The affected cornea is locally fibrotic with a more distinct vertical opacity near the central cornea. The mass was confirmed as a cyst by means of a fine-needle aspirate. The cyst and the corneal opacity may be a consequence of symblepharon or a prior surgical corneal-conjunctival transposition.

(Reproduced from *Veterinary Ocular Pathology: A Comparative Review*. Dubielzig, Ketring, McLellan, Albert. Elsevier Limited, 2010.)

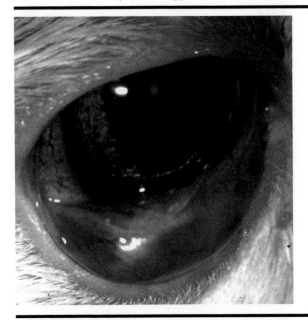

Figure 93
Conjunctival cyst
(2-year-old domestic shorthair)

As a kitten, this patient had an upper respiratory infection and conjunctivitis. The entire lower conjunctival cul-de-sac and inferior nictitans are distorted by a large cyst, confirmed by an acellular fine-needle aspirate.

(Reproduced from *Veterinary Ocular Pathology: A Comparative Review*. Dubielzig, Ketring, McLellan, Albert. Elsevier Limited, 2010.)

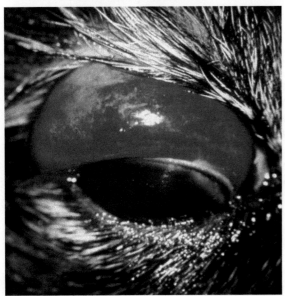

Figure 94
Subconjunctival hemorrhage/Hyphema
(3-year-old domestic shorthair)

Redness and swelling of the right eye were noted by the owners when their cat returned from out-of-doors. Blood beneath the dorsal conjunctiva distends the tissue beyond the lid margins, impairing lid function, and predisposing the surface to drying. Hyphema obscures intraocular detail. Trauma was the presumed etiology.

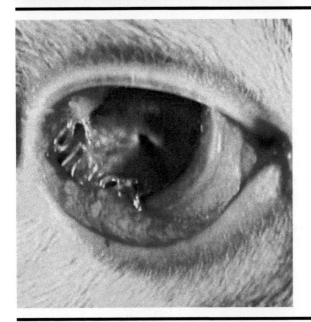

Figure 95
Thelaziasis
(3-year-old domestic shorthair)

A unilateral ocular discharge had been present for some time when owners noted a thread in the conjunctival cul-de-sac and presented the cat for removal of a foreign body. The conjunctiva is hyperemic and edematous. A thin, thread-like worm is coiled over the lateral aspect of the cornea. The nematode was identified as *Thelazia californiensis*.

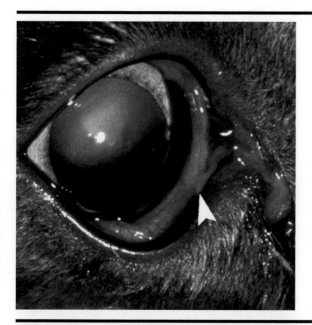

Figure 96
Dacryocystitis
(5-year-old domestic longhair)

A greenish ocular discharge had been present from the right eye for 6 months. The palpebral conjunctiva is chemotic and hyperemic. Mucopurulent discharge is present in the medial canthus. When a cannula was placed in the superior lacrimal punctum in an attempt to irrigate, a thick discharge came from the lower opening (*arrow*). No fluid or exudate exited the nares. Cytology identified a gram-negative rod, but culture results were negative.

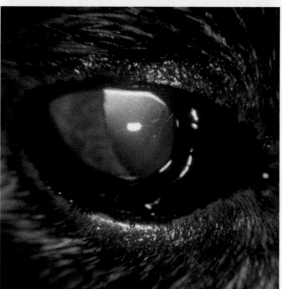

Figure 97
Conjunctival melanoma
(11-year-old domestic shorthair)

Progressive prominence and discoloration of the third eyelid were noted for 4 months prior to examination. A darkly pigmented third eyelid is accompanied by dark pigmentation and mild thickening of the bulbar and palpebral conjunctiva surrounding the globe. Intraocular structures are normal. An ipsilateral submandibular lymph node was also enlarged. Malignant melanoma was diagnosed following biopsy of the conjunctiva and fine-needle aspiration of the lymph node.

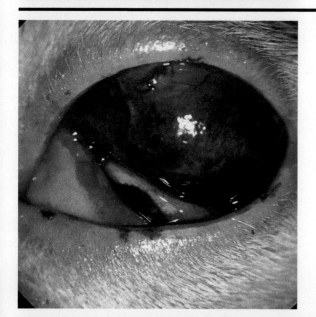

Figure 98
Conjunctival melanoma
(11-year-old DSH)

This mass had been gradually enlarging for several years. The heavily pigmented mass with its large surface vessels obscures the limbus superiorly. A small area of tan iris can be seen between the mass and the dark pupillary margin. On histopathology, this melanoma also extended intraocularly. The primary site of the neoplasm could not be determined.

SECTION V

Nictitating Membrane

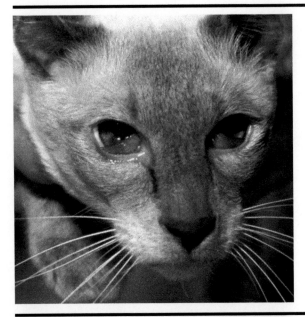

Figure 99
Idiopathic third eyelid protrusion/Haws syndrome
(4-year-old Siamese)

The only abnormality noted is the rather symmetrical protrusion of both third eyelids. Both retracted quickly following application of topical phenylephrine, indicating altered sympathetic innervation.

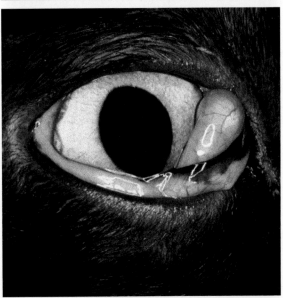

Figure 100
Prolapse of the gland of the third eyelid
(3-year-old Burmese)

The nictitans gland protrudes beyond the membrane's pigmented leading edge. The gland itself is normal despite the inadequacy of its connective tissue anchor.

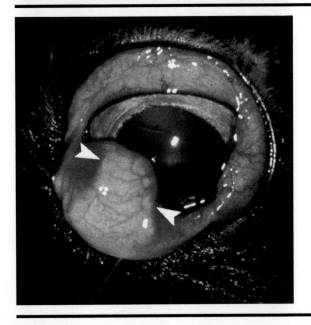

Figure 101
Everted third eyelid cartilage
(18-month-old Persian)

Presented for recurring conjunctivitis and protrusion of the third eyelid, this cat has moderate chemosis and mild hyperemia of the conjunctiva. The bulbar surface of the nictitating membrane and the cartilage can be seen between the arrows.

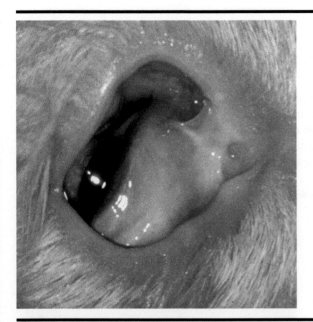

Figure 102
Symblepharon
(18-month-old domestic shorthair)

An abnormal adhesion is present from the superior lid to the palpebral surface of the third eyelid. The adhesion holds the nictitating membrane across the globe. An adhesion also covers the inferior nasolacrimal punctum, resulting in epiphora.

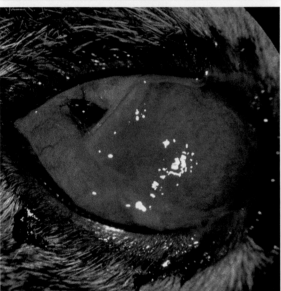

Figure 103
Abscess
(1-year-old domestic shorthair)

An acute onset of painful hyperemia and chemosis of the conjunctiva was followed by third eyelid swelling and prominence. A fine-needle aspirate was compatible with an infectious etiology. The initiating cause was never determined.

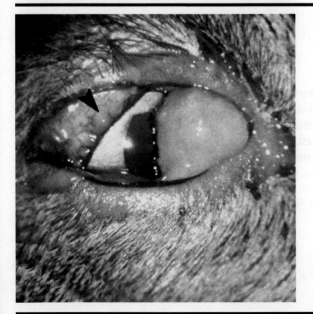

Figure 104
Eosinophilic conjunctivitis
(3-year-old domestic shorthair)

Owners watched as a mass enlarged over a 3-week period to obscure half the globe. A mucoid discharge and moderate conjunctival hyperemia accompany several perilimbal conjunctival nodules (*arrow*). The large flesh-colored mass near the medial canthus is the thickened margin of the third eyelid. Diagnosis was based on biopsy of the nictitans and cytology of a perilimbal conjunctival scraping.

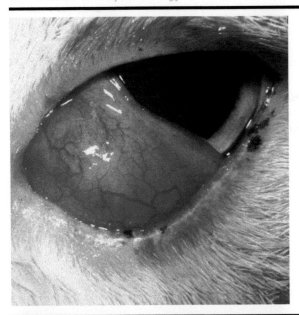

Figure 105
Fibrosarcoma
(15-year-old domestic shorthair)

Ocular problems were present for 2 months prior to this cat's examination. The nictitating membrane is enlarged and protrudes from its normal position. Palpation revealed a thickening of the entire membrane, narrowing to normal at its base. A FeLV test was negative. Histopathologic evaluation of the excised membrane was compatible with fibrosarcoma.

(Image courtesy of Nedim C. Buyukmihci, VMD, DACVO.)

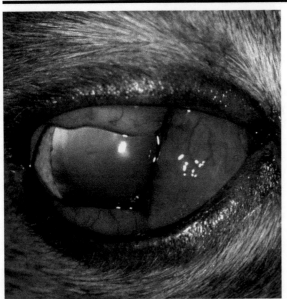

Figure 106
Squamous cell carcinoma
(18-year-old domestic shorthair)

Recently this exophthalmic globe, with moderate chemosis, developed a swollen prolapsed nictitans. Diagnosis was based on biopsy of the nictitans. The origin and extent of the tumor was not determined.

(Reproduced from *Veterinary Ocular Pathology: A Comparative Review*. Dubielzig, Ketring, McLellan, Albert. Elsevier Limited, 2010.)

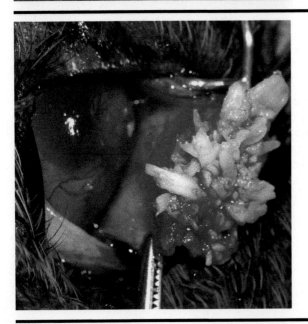

Figure 107
Squamous cell carcinoma
(13-year-old domestic longhair)

This cat was presented for evaluation of a progressively enlarging mass arising from the bulbar surface of the third eyelid. The nictitans has been everted to demonstrate the white finger-like projections that characterize the tumor. Corneal vascularization and scattered surface opacities are secondary to long-standing herpesvirus infection and eosinophilic keratitis. Squamous cell carcinoma was diagnosed on biopsy of the third eyelid mass. Interestingly, a firm subconjunctival mass in the inferior cul-de-sac of the opposite eye was diagnosed as a desmoplastic squamous cell carcinoma.

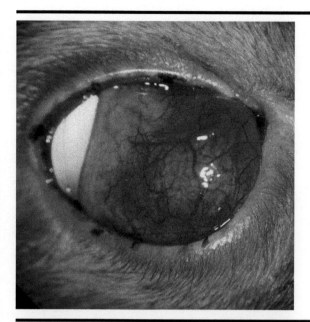

Figure 108
Lymphoma
(5-year-old domestic shorthair)

The third eyelid features a large well-delineated mass, swollen above the less hyperemic marginal tissue. The cat showed no subjective signs of pain. No other ocular abnormalities were noted. A fine-needle aspirate revealed neoplastic lymphocytes.

(Reproduced from *Veterinary Ocular Pathology: A Comparative Review*. Dubielzig, Ketring, McLellan, Albert. Elsevier Limited, 2010.)

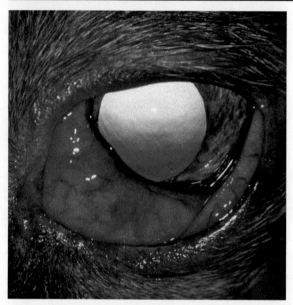

Figure 109
Plasmacytoma
(16-year-old Siamese)

The third eyelid is mildly prolapsed and diffusely swollen. Ventral conjunctiva is chemotic and extends above the eyelid margin. A fine-needle aspirate included a population of highly pleomorphic and multinucleated round cells compatible with a plasmacytoma. The red tapetal reflection is normal in this color-dilute breed.

SECTION VI

Cornea

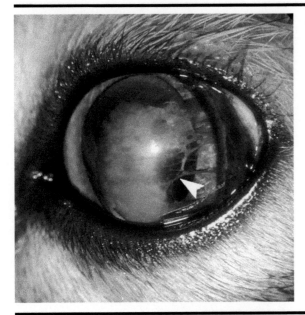

Figure 110
Persistent pupillary membranes (PPM)
(6-month-old domestic shorthair)

Pigmented strands (*arrow*) similar in color to that of the iris originate from the iris collarette and attach to the corneal endothelium. The PPMs create a web-like network near the inner corneal surface. Corneal edema decreases the visibility of the mottled endothelial pigmentation.

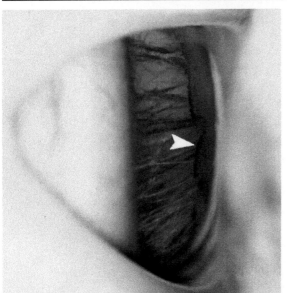

Figure 111
Persistent pupillary membranes (PPM)
(6-month-old domestic longhair)

A lateral view of the right eye shows numerous pigmented strands originating from the iris face, spanning the anterior chamber and attaching to the inner corneal surface. The result is a dense, pigmented layer (*arrow*) created at the endothelial level. The clinical consequences included a large axial area of corneal edema and fibrosis.

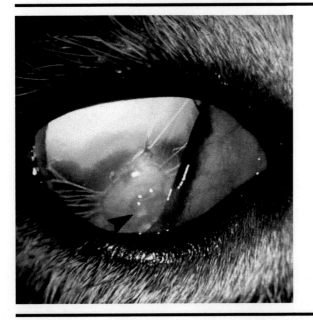

Figure 112
Persistent pupillary membranes/Bullous keratitis
(1.5-year-old domestic shorthair)

The pupil has been dilated as part of the initial examination, obscuring the origin of the PPMs. Multiple pigmented strands, highlighted by the tapetal reflection, insert at the corneal endothelial level. Over a period of time, secondary corneal edema has progressed to include multiple subepithelial fluid bullae (*arrow*).

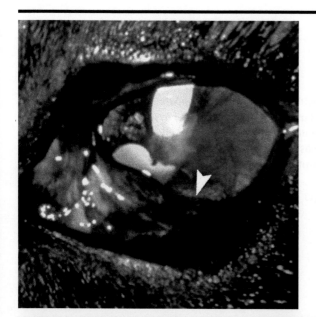

Figure 113
Adherent leukoma
(adult domestic shorthair)

This stray cat was presented for evaluation of excessive tearing and a cloudy central cornea. The nictitating membrane (*arrow*) is diffusely pigmented and permanently prolapsed because of adhesions between the bulbar and palpebral conjunctiva. The axial cornea is scarred, with attachment of the iris to the endothelial surface. Iris atrophy is also present to the left of the scar. The lacrimal puncta were obliterated by conjunctival adhesions, accounting for the epiphora. Ulceration secondary to feline herpesvirus infection was blamed for the symblepharon. The central scar implies a previously perforated corneal ulcer.

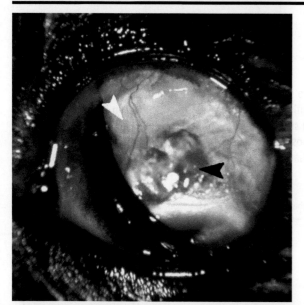

Figure 114
Terriens marginal corneal degeneration
(9-year-old domestic longhair)

The vascularization, white discoloration, and irregular contours of the corneas first started in the left eye 3 years prior to this photograph. Abnormalities were confined to the cornea, which was edematous (*white arrow*), vascularized, and thinner than normal (*black arrow*). The epithelium is intact but elevated by diffuse white lipid deposits. Diagnosis was confirmed by histopathology.

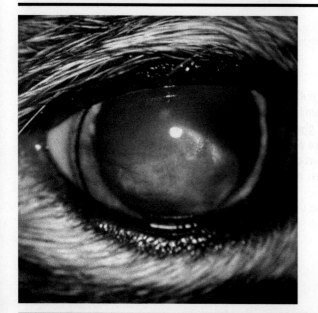

Figure 115
Corneal degeneration
(16-year-old domestic shorthair)

This patient had a history of ocular trauma, although details of the injury were unknown. The white ill-defined central opacity has the granular, refractile appearance of a stromal lipid infiltrate. Vascularization of the cornea is also present. A distinct white circular flash artifact is present at the dorsal margin of the opacity.

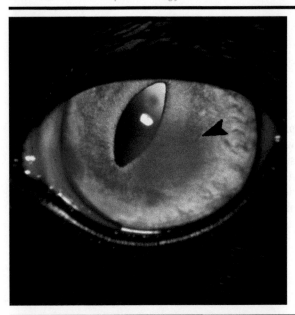

Figure 116
Florida spots
(2-year-old domestic shorthair)

Multiple poorly demarcated opacities are apparent in the temporal (*arrow*) and nasal corneal quadrants of this otherwise asymptomatic cat. This nonprogressive condition is recognized more often in companion animals within the southeastern United States. The causative agent or mechanism has yet to be determined.

(Image courtesy of Art J. Quinn, DVM, DACVO.)

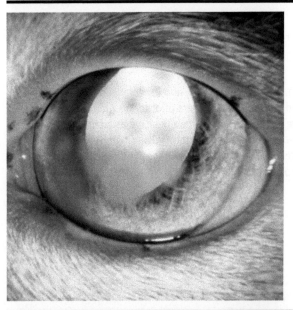

Figure 117
Florida spots
(5.5-year-old domestic shorthair)

The cat showed no signs of discomfort or vision impairment associated with this bilateral condition. Multiple gray-white opacities can be seen in the superficial corneal stroma, the light color more easily appreciated overlying the medial iris. Those lesions overlying the pupillary region appear dark as they obscure the background tapetal reflection. A causative agent was not identified.

(Image courtesy of Kathleen P. Barrie DVM, MS, DACVO.)

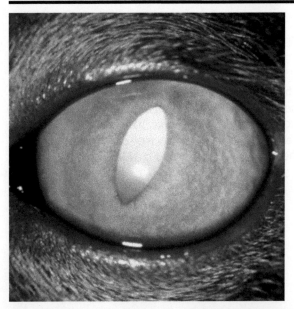

Figure 118
Mucopolysaccharidosis VI
(6-month-old domestic shorthair)

The iris appears dull and relatively featureless because of a diffuse corneal haze. On retroillumination, the corneal clouding appears granular, owing to accumulation of glycosaminoglycans within vacuolated keratocytes. Affected animals also have widely separated palpebral fissures and thickened eyelids. The diagnosis was confirmed by a positive blue toluidine spot test, which signifies an excess of mucopolysaccharide in urine.

(Image courtesy of Art J. Quinn, DVM, DACVO.)

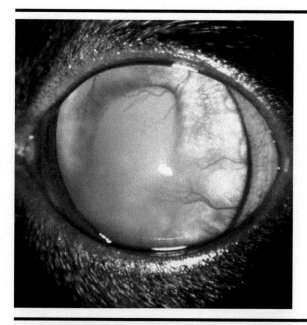

Figure 119
Relapsing polychondritis
(3-year-old Siamese)

Cloudy corneas had been present for several months when owners also noticed progressive curling of the ear tips. Neither eye appeared painful, despite mild conjunctival hyperemia. The corneal surface is diffusely hazy, with focal superficial stromal opacities and vascularization. The array of clinical signs and histopathologic findings were compatible with an inflammatory connective tissue disease, relapsing polychondritis (RPC). Greater than half the human patients with RPC develop ocular signs, including scleritis, conjunctivitis, keratoconjunctivitis sicca, and keratitis.

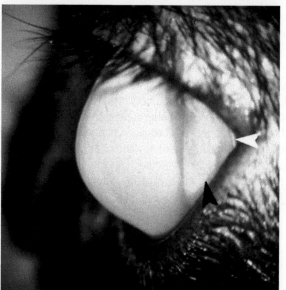

Figure 120
Keratoconus/Corneal edema
(8-year-old domestic shorthair)

This bilateral condition had progressively worsened over the past 6 months. The cat was comfortable and showed no vision deficit despite the severe corneal edema that alters the corneal contour. The intraocular pressure was normal. The limbus (*white arrow*) and the iris (*black arrow*) are marked for orientation. Refer to Figure 5 for a photograph of normal corneal curvature.

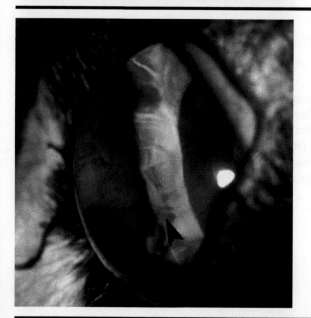

Figure 121
Keratoconus
(4-year-old domestic shorthair)

This cat developed a severe anterior uveitis and bullous keratitis of undetermined cause 20 months prior to the photograph. The original problems improved with medication. The cornea subsequently thinned, developing an exaggerated curvature. The drainage angle (*arrow*) appears abnormal because of altered refraction by the cornea. Intraocular pressure and vision remained normal.

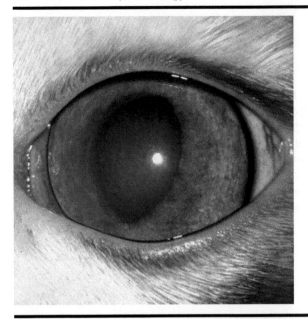

Figure 122
Manx dystrophy
(8-month-old Manx)

This patient demonstrates the early stages of this rare, inherited, and progressive corneal disorder. The central cornea appears blue because of stromal edema, but milder edema is also present peripherally. With time, the edema and corneal opacification worsen. Large coalescing intrastromal bullae and secondary superficial vascularization characterize the more advanced stages of the disease.

(Image courtesy of Steven I. Bistner, DVM, DACVO.)

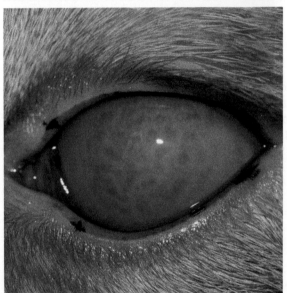

Figure 123
Congenital corneal edema
(3-year-old domestic shorthair)

The referring veterinarian first noted localized corneal cloudiness in both eyes when this cat was 4 months of age. The cloudiness increased to its current level over the subsequent 18 months. The entire corneal surface appears blue, with a stippled character suggestive of corneal endothelial dysfunction. Intraocular examination, performed at an earlier stage of the problem, was normal. Intraocular pressure has remained normal. This cat retained a dazzle reflex and excellent motion detection, but near vision was compromised.

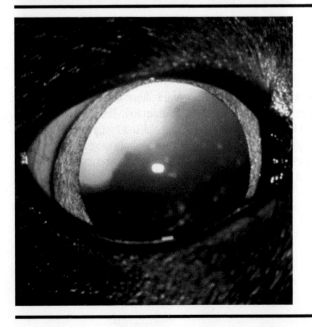

Figure 124
Herpetic keratitis—Punctate
(18-month-old domestic shorthair)

This cat was presented for evaluation of corneal opacity and vascularization in the left eye, subsequently diagnosed as eosinophilic keratitis. The photograph is of the opposite right cornea. Multiple punctate epithelial opacities, stained positively with fluorescein, can be seen against the dark nontapetal background. Notice the lack of conjunctival hyperemia. The punctate lesions cleared quickly in response to a topical antiviral agent.

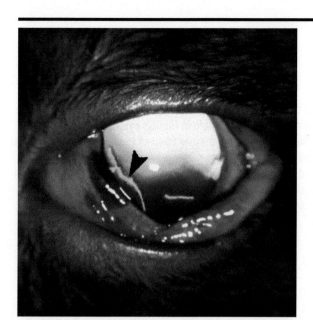

Figure 125
Herpetic keratitis—Dendritic
(18-month-old domestic shorthair)

Bilateral blepharospasm and tearing led the owners to present this cat for examination. The conjunctiva is hyperemic and chemotic. The prominent third eyelid is typical of a painful eye. Linear pathognomonic dendritic ulcers can be seen at the arrow. The lesions cleared when treated with a topical antiviral drug.

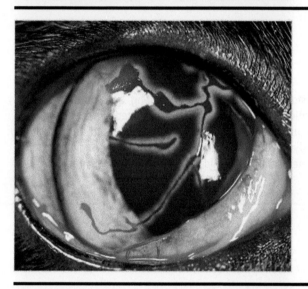

Figure 126
Herpetic keratitis—Dendritic
(4-year-old domestic shorthair)

This dendritic ulcer is stained with both fluorescein and rose bengal, highlighting the linear, branching features that are pathognomonic for herpesvirus infection. The areas of green fluorescein retention indicate loss of the entire epithelial layer, with exposure of the superficial stroma. The pink to red color of the rose bengal vital stain identifies earlier cytopathic effects of herpesvirus infection, i.e., devitalized or necrotic epithelial cells rather than complete loss of the epithelial layer. The bright white opacities are flash artifacts.

(Image courtesy of David T. Ramsey, DVM, MS, DACVO.)

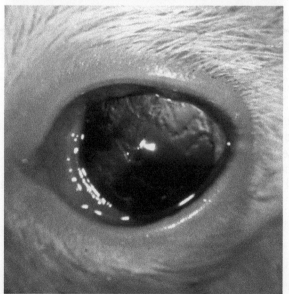

Figure 127
Herpetic keratitis—Early geographic
(1-year-old domestic shorthair)

The left eye is representative of a bilateral problem in this young cat. Multiple linear superficial ulcers are present and are most easily seen against the blue tapetal background. Although some opacities do not stain positively, a large area of fluorescein retention can be seen extending between the leading edge of the third eyelid and the central cornea. Dendrites in this region have coalesced, completely disrupting the epithelial surface.

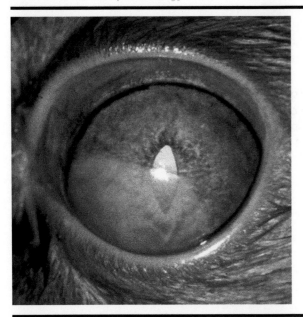

Figure 128
Herpetic ulcer—Geographic
(8-month-old Persian)

This cat had been treated for a herpetic keratitis in the right eye for 2 months when he was presented with acute pain in the left eye. Severe blepharospasm diminished following application of topical anesthetic to facilitate examination. Conjunctival hyperemia accompanies a large fluorescein-stained superficial ulcer in the ventral cornea. Concurrent signs of anterior uveitis include miosis, subtle aqueous flare, iris swelling, and decreased intraocular pressure. All signs quickly subsided with topical antiviral therapy.

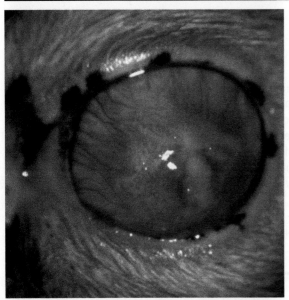

Figure 129
Herpetic keratitis—Geographic
(6-year-old exotic shorthair)

This cat had a history of squinting, excessive tearing, and corneal ulceration of 3 months duration. Both eyes were similarly affected. Severe superficial vascularization is present. The axial cornea is edematous and stains positively with fluorescein dye. Although the immunofluorescent antibody test for herpesvirus was negative, lesions did respond to topical antiviral medication.

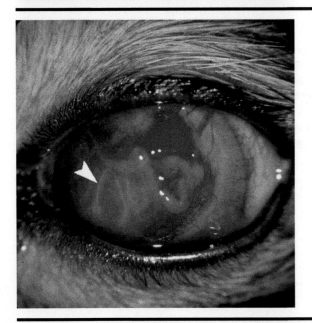

Figure 130
Herpetic keratitis—Geographic/Bullous
(1-year-old Somali)

This kitten is one of a litter of three, all demonstrating notable corneal disease. Thickened, hyperplastic epithelium creates a vermiform ridge in the axial cornea. Corneal vascularization is prominent, especially dorsally where a raised granulation bed can be seen. Large fluid bullae (*arrow*) overlie the edematous central cornea. Dendritic ulcerations were present in the opposite eye.

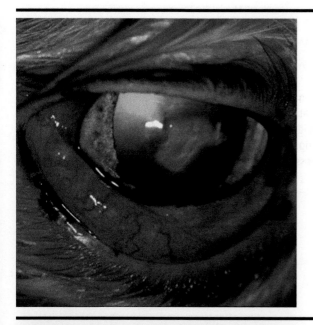

Figure 131
Herpetic keratitis—Recrudescence
(8-year-old exotic shorthair)

First diagnosed with feline herpesvirus-1 (FHV-1) as a 5-year old, this cat relapsed 3 years later after treatment for asthma with oral corticosteroids. Conjunctival hyperemia and chemosis accompany a central irregularly shaped fluorescein-positive geographic ulcer.

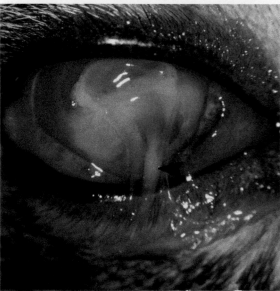

Figure 132
Mycoplasma
(16-year-old domestic shorthair)

Previously diagnosed with herpetic keratitis, this cat also had a long history of upper respiratory disease. One week prior to this photograph, he received a cortisone injection and is now being treated with an antibiotic ointment. Marked conjunctival hyperemia accompanies ulceration and severe keratomalacia ("melting") of the central cornea. Intense corneal edema surrounds a slightly clearer center that suggests greater stromal thinning. Prominent corneal vascularization can be seen temporally. What appears to be mucus overlying the central cornea and lower lid margin (*arrow*) is actually necrotic stroma. *Mycoplasma* spp was cultured from the axial cornea.

(Reproduced from *Veterinary Ocular Pathology: A Comparative Review*. Dubielzig, Ketring, McLellan, Albert. Elsevier Limited, 2010.)

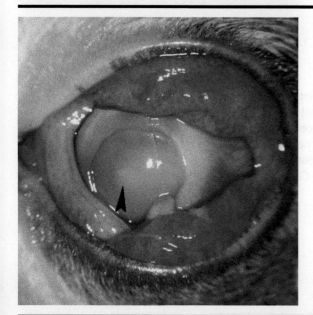

Figure 133
Mycoplasma
(3-year-old domestic shorthair)

This stray cat developed conjunctivitis after its arrival at an animal shelter. Treatment consisted of a triple antibiotic-corticosteroid ointment. Severely chemotic and hyperemic conjunctiva join with a prominent third eyelid to frame the edematous, vascularized cornea. A circular stromal ulcer, with a cream-colored cellular infiltrate (*arrow*) at its center, occupies the axial cornea. *Mycoplasma* spp was cultured from the ulcer.

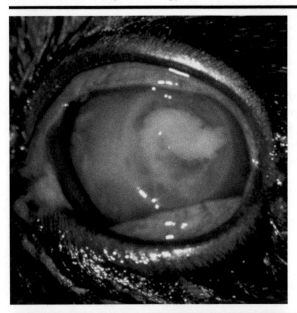

Figure 134
Bacterial keratitis/Staphylococcus
(3-month-old Persian)

The conjunctiva is moderately chemotic and hyperemic. Deep and superficial corneal vascularization and diffuse edema are present. A large circular stromal ulcer is evident beneath a thick discharge adhering to the corneal surface. The anterior chamber is difficult to see, but the pupil is miotic and the intraocular pressure is greatly reduced. *Staphylococcus* spp was cultured from the ulcer.

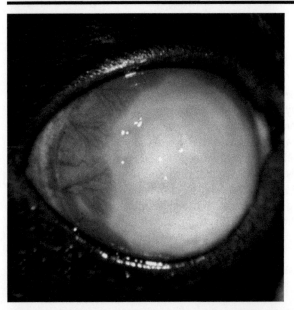

Figure 135
Bacterial keratitis/Pseudomonas
(8.5-year-old domestic shorthair)

This cat was being treated for bilateral herpetic keratitis and toxoplasma-induced uveitis with topical antiviral drugs and systemic and topical corticosteroids. He presented with a 2-day history of intense ocular pain and cloudy corneas. The anterior segment cannot be visualized because of severe keratomalacia and superficial corneal vascularization. The left eye was similarly, but less severely, affected. Intraocular pressure was markedly reduced in both eyes. A pure culture of *Pseudomonas aeruginosa* was isolated from both corneas.

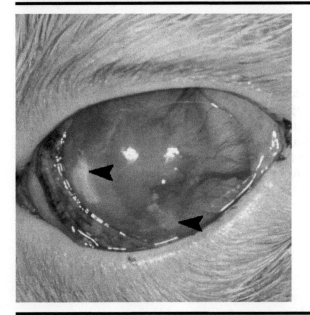

Figure 136
Mycotic keratitis
(8-year-old domestic shorthair)

A variety of antibiotic-corticosteroid ophthalmic preparations had been used to treat a persistent corneal ulcer of 3 weeks' duration. Superficial vessels surround a large central superficial ulcer. The cornea is diffusely edematous, with inflammatory cell infiltrates appearing as yellowish plaques (*arrows*). The axial defect retained fluorescein. Culture and cytology of the ulcer margin identified *Candida albicans* as the causative agent.

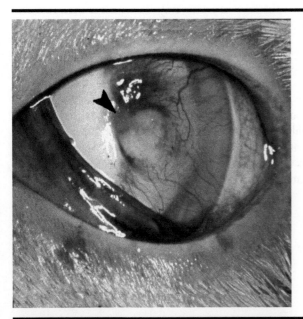

Figure 137
Mycotic keratitis
(8-year-old domestic shorthair)

Subjective signs of pain had increased over the last 10 days, during which a boric acid flush had been used to manage the cat's ocular discharge. Pain was manifest by blepharospasm and protrusion of the third eyelid. The conjunctiva is moderately hyperemic. The temporal half of the cornea is superficially vascularized, with vessels encircling a paraxial stromal ulcer. The margins of the ulcer are necrotic (*arrow*). A moderate anterior uveitis accompanied the corneal lesion, though signs are difficult to visualize in the photo. Hemolytic *Staphylococcus* spp and *Aspergillus fumigatus* were cultured from the margins of the defect.

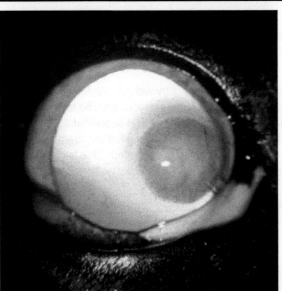

Figure 138
Mycobacterial keratitis
(young adult domestic shorthair)

The duration of the corneal opacity and the presence of additional lesions in this indoor/outdoor cat were unknown. No discomfort was associated with a smooth, elevated, well-vascularized subepithelial and intrastromal granuloma located in the peripheral cornea. Acid fast bacilli within the tissue were identified as *Mycobacterium intracellulare*. The character of the granuloma suggested an early stage of infection.

(Image courtesy of Richard Malik, DVsc, PhD, DipVetAn, MvetClinStud.)

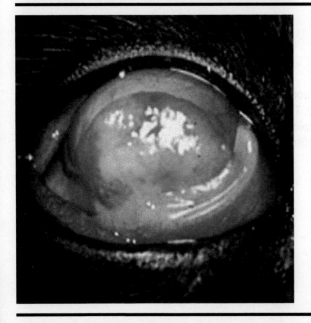

Figure 139
Mycobacterial keratitis
(6-year-old domestic longhair)

This outdoor cat had a history of prior corneal trauma and then a 5-month progression of corneal infiltration. A large granuloma effaces two-thirds of the right cornea, obscuring intraocular detail. The left eye and the cat's general health were unaffected. The cat was FIV positive and FeLV negative. Culture of the corneal lesion was unrewarding. On histopathology, acid fast bacilli were found within macrophages in the deep stromal infiltrate. The organism was identified as a novel *Mycobacterium* spp by PCR amplification.

(Image courtesy of Christina McCowan, BVSc, BSc (Hons), MACVS, PhD, Honorary Fellow Veterinary Ophthalmic Pathology: Novel fastidious Mycobacterium causing lepromatous lesions of the skin, subcutis, cornea, and conjunctiva of cats living in Victoria, Australia. *Clin Microbiol* 46(2): 618–626, 2007.)

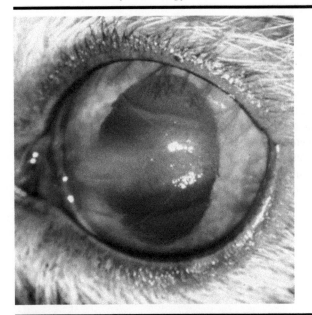

Figure 140
Superficial ulcer/Trigeminal and facial nerve paresis
(13-year-old domestic shorthair)

This cat had a history of a corneal ulcer in the left eye following the surgical removal of an oral squamous cell carcinoma. Superficial corneal vessels are present, most notably in the dorsal quadrant. A horizontally oriented ellipse of dull, roughened axial cornea stains positively with fluorescein. Corneal sensitivity and blink response were poor. The Schirmer tear test measured 5 mm/min. The location and shape of the corneal lesion are often seen with lagophthalmos.

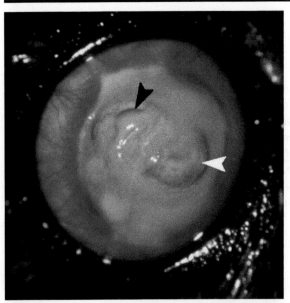

Figure 141
Bullous keratitis
(5-year-old Persian)

One month prior to presentation, this cat survived a house fire, suffering smoke inhalation and developing bilateral corneal ulcers. The left eye had healed without incident. Diffuse corneal edema and superficial vascularization are still present in the right cornea. Multiple stromal bullae (*black arrow*) create an irregular central corneal contour. One large bulla is fluorescein positive (*white arrow*).

(Reproduced from *Veterinary Ocular Pathology: A Comparative Review*. Dubielzig, Ketring, McLellan, Albert. Elsevier Limited, 2010.)

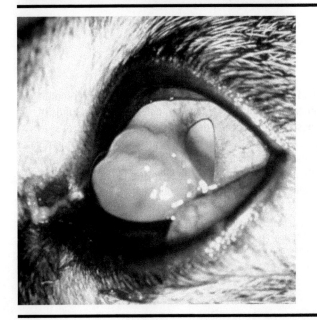

Figure 142
Bullous keratopathy
(2.5-year-old domestic shorthair)

The axial cornea protrudes anteriorly because of extreme stromal edema that developed acutely. The conjunctiva is chemotic and hyperemic, accompanying a mild anterior uveitis. Note the lack of corneal vascularization and surrounding corneal edema. Bacterial culture was negative.

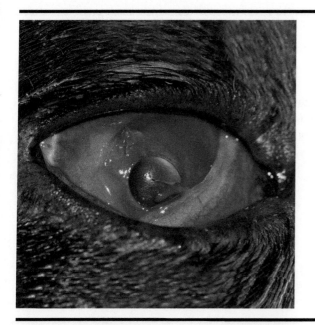

Figure 143
Descemetocele
(young adult domestic shorthair)

No history was known for this patient presented by an animal rescue group. Conjunctival hyperemia accompanies a prominent third eyelid. The corneal surface is edematous, with active superficial vascularization temporally. The axial cornea is deeply ulcerated. A slight difference in corneal opacity highlights the boundary between the peripheral cornea and the stromal defect. A well-defined descemetocele at the ulcer's center provides a clear view of the tapetal reflection. Loose epithelium is present near the upper margin of the descemetocele, while a strand of mucus overlies its lower edge.

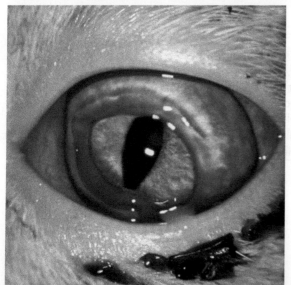

Figure 144
Descemetocele
(young adult domestic shorthair)

The owner found this stray and presented him immediately for evaluation. The right eye had a large axial staphyloma. This left eye has a large central descemetocele through which the iris and pupil can easily be seen. The cornea at the margins of the descemetocele is edematous. Bacterial cultures were negative.

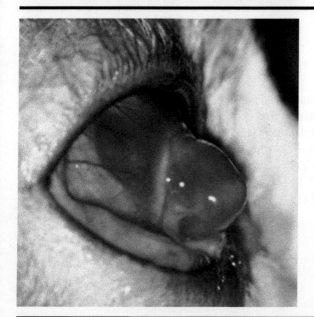

Figure 145
Iris prolapse
(10.5-year-old domestic shorthair)

This patient's cornea deteriorated over a 72-hour period following the appearance of a superficial corneal ulcer. The conjunctiva appears chemotic and hyperemic. Superficial vessels extend from the limbus to the axial cornea. Iris protrudes through a perforated central ulcer and is covered by a fibrinohemorrhagic clot. The anterior chamber is extremely shallow.

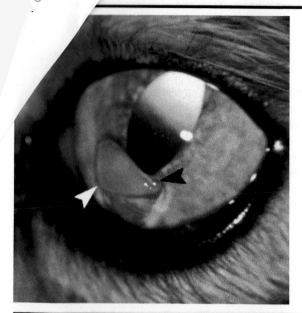

Figure 146
Corneal laceration
(10-year-old domestic longhair)

Acute blepharospasm and tearing were seen following a cat fight. The apex (*white arrow*) of a triangular flap of edematous corneal tissue is displaced dorsally from its origin at 6 o'clock, while its base remains attached axially (*black arrow*).

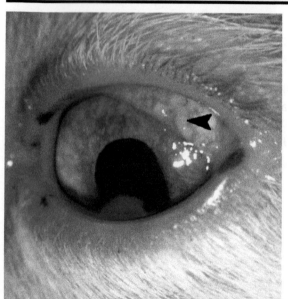

Figure 147
Eosinophilic keratitis/Herpetic keratitis
(18-month-old domestic longhair)

Eight months prior to this photograph, the cat was diagnosed with and successfully treated for herpetic keratitis in the right eye. A large superficial ulcer in the ventral left cornea retains stain. The raised yellow plaques (*arrow*) in the perilimbal bulbar conjunctiva appeared white and grainy prior to fluorescein application, consistent with an early stage of eosinophilic keratitis.

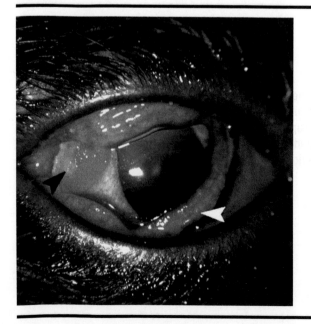

Figure 148
Eosinophilic keratitis/Herpetic keratitis
(3.5-year-old domestic longhair)

This was a bilateral condition that developed in conjunction with an upper respiratory infection of 6 weeks' duration. Oral and topical antibiotics had been administered during that time. Focal gritty deposits present on the hyperemic conjunctiva and nictitans (*white arrow*) lend a subtly nodular appearance to the affected surfaces. The temporal cornea is ulcerated. Cellular infiltrates and the same gritty white precipitates (*black arrow*) found in the conjunctiva contribute to the lesion's dull, matte appearance.

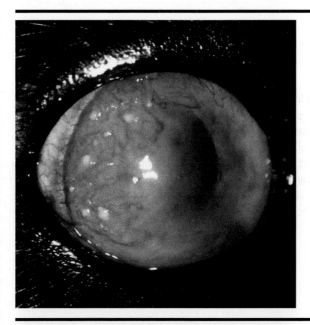

Figure 149
Eosinophilic keratitis
(7-year-old domestic longhair)

This patient was adopted from a shelter at 4–5 weeks of age. No ocular problems had been noted prior to 2 weeks ago, when both eyes became red and cloudy. Neither eye appeared painful. No improvement had been noted with use of a topical antibiotic ointment. The temporal cornea is edematous, with actively branching vessels within the superficial stroma and multiple white-raised plaques scattered across the affected surface. Corneal vascularization extends into the dorsal and ventral cornea. A bright light artifact is present at the leading edge of the vessels. Examination of a scraping of a surface plaque revealed a variety of inflammatory cells, including eosinophils. The opposite eye was less severely affected.

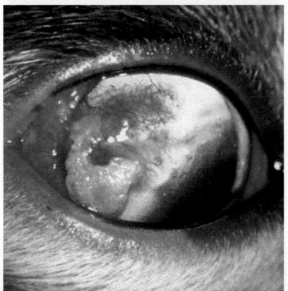

Figure 150
Eosinophilic keratitis
(3-year-old domestic shorthair)

There had been a 3-month history of recurring ulcers and vascularization in both corneas. Response to a topical antibiotic-corticosteroid ointment had been poor. Both eyes were similarly affected at the time of examination. The hyperemic lids were attributed to neomycin sensitivity. The conjunctiva is moderately hyperemic. Prominent blood vessels surround a large white superficial plaque, its grainy surface raised above the surrounding tissue. Smaller plaques are present on the conjunctiva. A fluorescein dye test was negative.

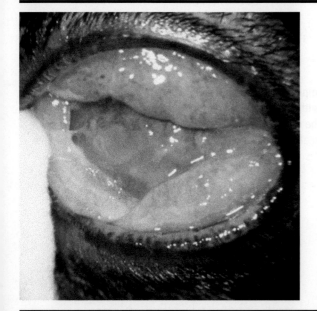

Figure 151
Eosinophilic keratitis/Conjunctivitis
(5-year-old domestic shorthair)

Despite 3 years of treatment with topical antibiotics, the left eye had failed to respond to therapy and was now blind. The palpebral conjunctiva and third eyelid are hyperemic and markedly thickened. The exposed surfaces are friable and bleed easily when manipulated. The corneal surface is irregular; plaques of flesh-colored tissue within the superficial cornea are well vascularized. Diagnosis was based on biopsy of corneal and conjunctival tissues.

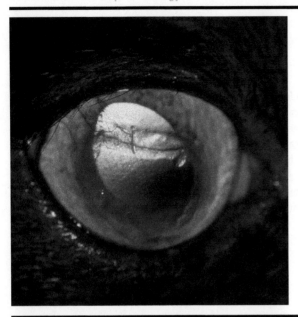

Figure 152
Corneal sequestration
(3-year-old Himalayan)

This patient had a lifelong history of ocular discharge and intermittent but self-limiting bouts of squinting affecting the right eye. The most recent episode began 3 weeks ago, persisting despite a week-long regimen of topical antibacterial. The central cornea is ulcerated, with poorly adherent epithelium outlined dorsally by the tapetal reflection. That same reflection is obscured in the lower half of the pupil by ill-defined bronzing of the stroma, indicative of early sequestrum formation. Superficial vessels extend from the dorsal limbus to the ulcer site.

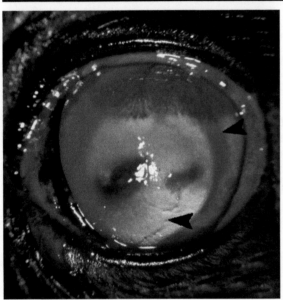

Figure 153
Corneal sequestration/Herpetic keratitis
(9-month-old Persian)

Three months prior to the photograph, this cat was diagnosed with an upper respiratory infection, bilateral ulcerative keratitis, and brown discoloration of the corneas. Both eyes are still affected. The cornea is diffusely edematous and vascularized superiorly. The edge of a large unstained ulcer is present at the arrows. Two focal areas of brown discoloration are present within the ulcer. The Schirmer tear test in both eyes was 5 mm/min.

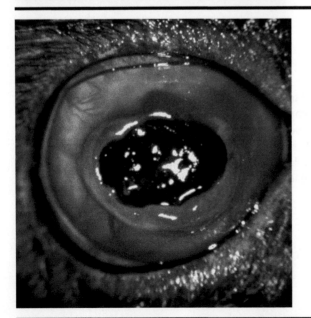

Figure 154
Corneal sequestration/Anterior uveitis
(14-year-old Persian)

History was incomplete in this case. The cat demonstrated severe blepharospasm with miosis and decreased intraocular pressure. The large black plaque in the central cornea has an elevated, loosened edge. The surrounding corneal stroma is edematous and infiltrated by superficial and deep blood vessels.

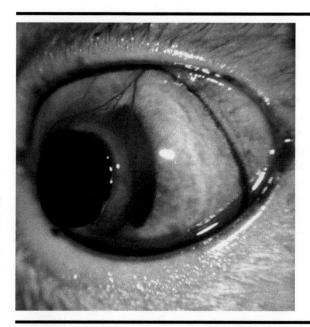

Figure 155
Corneal sequestration
(4.5-year-old Himalayan)

This cat developed bilateral corneal ulcers 6 months prior to the photograph. Both eyes are again similarly affected. A large black plaque is clearly elevated above the underlying tissue and is surrounded by edematous, vascularized stroma. One month later, the plaque spontaneously sloughed.

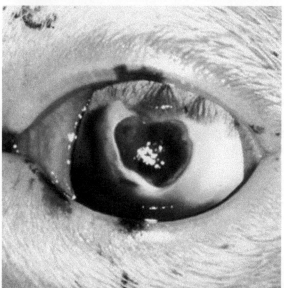

Figure 156
Corneal foreign body
(3-year-old domestic shorthair)

Owners noted their cat squinting for 2 weeks. Plant material appears as a darkly colored, elevated plaque in the central cornea, with edematous edges and a vascularized upper border. The foreign body was removed with a flat spatula following topical anesthesia.

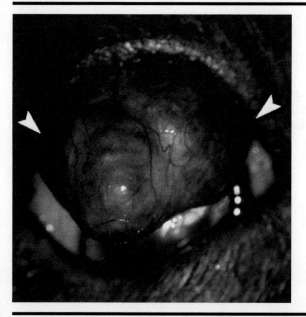

Figure 157
Staphyloma
(6-year-old domestic shorthair)

The owner noticed a black mass growing over the eye for a period of several months. A large, darkly pigmented, irregular subconjunctival mass (between the *arrows*) originates superior to the limbus and obscures a portion of the adjacent cornea. A melanoma was suspected and the globe was enucleated. The histopathologic diagnosis was a staphyloma. The initiating factor was not determined.

(Reproduced from *Veterinary Ocular Pathology: A Comparative Review*. Dubielzig, Ketring, McLellan, Albert. Elsevier Limited, 2010.)

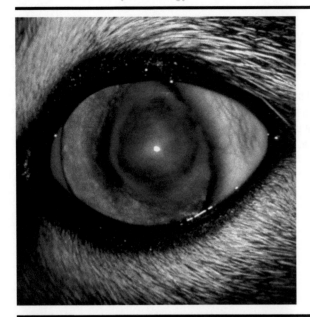

Figure 158
Staphyloma/Adherent leukoma
(8-year-old domestic shorthair)

This was a comfortable eye with no signs of active inflammation. The blue-gray appearance of the cornea is a consequence of scarring and adhesion of the iris to the cornea. The cornea at the scar's center is thin and protrudes anteriorly. Severe corneal disease and anterior uveitis must have preceded this condition.

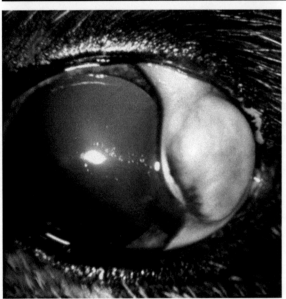

Figure 159
Staphyloma
(7-year-old domestic shorthair)

The owner reported that the appearance of this eye had remained unchanged for several years. The globe's contour is distorted by herniation of the iris and ciliary body into an area of thinned, outwardly stretched sclera. The iridocorneal drainage angle adjacent to the elevation was closed by peripheral anterior synechiae.

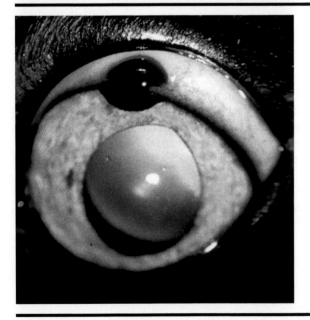

Figure 160
Limbal melanocytoma
(10-year-old domestic shorthair)

This benign tumor originates over the superior sclera and extends into the adjacent corneal stroma but is causing no active inflammation or discomfort. An unrelated lens luxation creates an aphakic crescent visible within the ventral pupil.

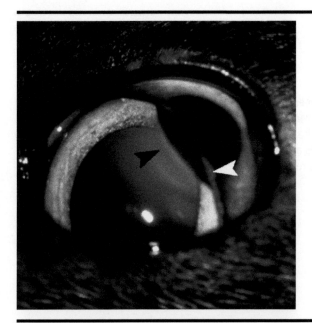

Figure 161
Limbal melanocytoma
(19-year-old domestic shorthair)

The duration of this lesion was unknown. The *white arrow* marks the limbus. Superiorly, a black mass elevated beneath the conjunctiva extends into the corneal stroma. The axial margin of the mass has a white, granular appearance, suggestive of a lipid infiltrate (*black arrow*). These slow-growing tumors originate from the pigmented cells of the scleral shelf.

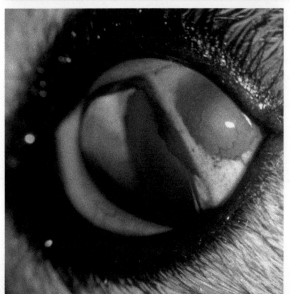

Figure 162
Limbal melanocytoma
(6-year-old domestic shorthair)

The owner was unaware of an ocular problem until the referring veterinarian pointed out a raised pigmented mass in the lateral sclera during a routine health maintenance visit. At examination 2 weeks later, a raised, well-defined pigmented mass overlies the sclera, beneath the temporal conjunctiva. Pigmented tissue also extends into the adjacent cornea but spares the perilimbal sclera, in contrast to the patient in Figure 161. The iridocorneal angle was unaffected gonioscopically. The photo is taken at an angle, with the dark pupil appearing near the tumor site, the yellowish iris seen on the opposite side of the eye, and the third eyelid margin visible as a pale curvilinear area medially.

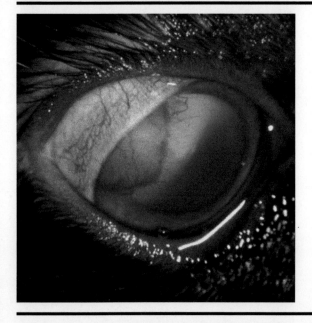

Figure 163
Neuroblastic tumor
(4-year-old Himalayan)

This lesion developed quickly over a 2-week period. A tan to pink mass is present within the deep corneal layers, extending into the adjacent sclera. The overlying cornea is vascularized. The iris was grossly spared based on gonioscopic examination. The tumor was believed to be metastatic and neuroblastic, although the precise origin of the tumor was never determined.

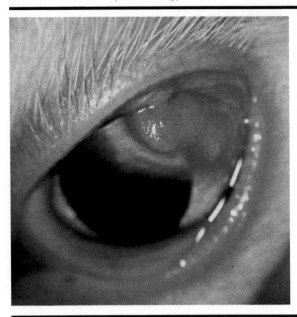

Figure 164
Squamous cell carcinoma
(8-year-old domestic shorthair)

This mass had been slowly progressing from the limbal cornea with minimal detectable involvement of the sclera and only mild conjunctival hyperemia and chemosis. The white-elevated mass was smooth and demonstrated only thin deep vessels and little superficial vascularization. The diagnosis was based on biopsy results.

(Image courtesy of David T. Ramsey, DVM, MS, DACVO.)

SECTION VII

Anterior Uvea

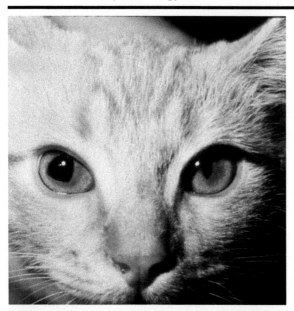

Figure 165
Iris coloboma
(juvenile domestic shorthair)

A temporal notch-like defect in the right pupil compromises its response to light. This developmental defect must be differentiated from pupillary abnormalities caused by neurologic deficits (see Figure 169).

(Image courtesy of Art J. Quinn, DVM, DACVO.)

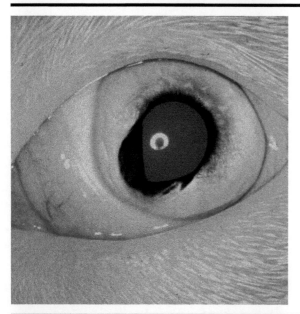

Figure 166
Iris coloboma
(1-year-old domestic shorthair)

An abnormally shaped pupil led to this cat's examination. The iris stroma, embryologically derived from mesoderm, is poorly developed at the ventronasal pupillary margin. The posterior pigmented layers of the iris that arise from neuroectoderm are present but incomplete. The pupillary light response is essentially normal elsewhere but limited at the coloboma site.

(Reproduced from *Veterinary Ocular Pathology: A Comparative Review*. Dubielzig, Ketring, McLellan, Albert. Elsevier Limited, 2010.)

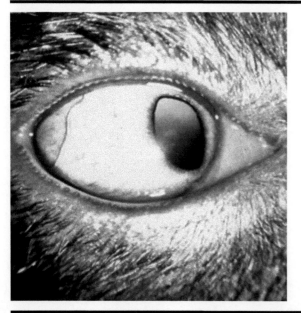

Figure 167
Corectopia
(4-month-old Burmese)

The owner commented on her kitten's cross-eyed appearance during a health maintenance examination. The third eyelid is prominent and mildly hyperemic. The pupil tilts along it vertical axis and is offset nasally. Poor iridal response to mydriatics limited evaluation of the lens and fundus, but gross abnormalities were not apparent. The left eye was also affected. At first glance, the anomaly mimics the convergent strabismus of the Siamese breed.

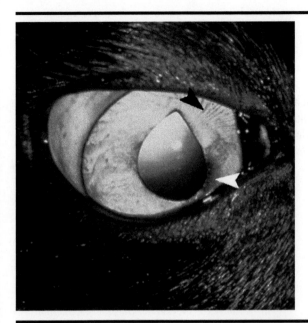

Figure 168
Dyscoria
(1-year-old domestic shorthair)

This cat had a history of seizures. The pupil is irregular, with a reverse D shape and no response to light. The nasal iris is dark in color (*white arrow*); radial bands appear in other iris quadrants (*black arrow*). The left pupil was a small vertical slit that failed to dilate normally. The cause of the dyscoria and seizures was not established.

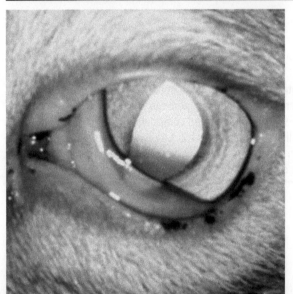

Figure 169
D-shaped pupil
(6-year-old domestic shorthair)

Lack of innervation by the temporal short ciliary nerve is the presumed cause of the abnormal pupil shape. The temporal iris remains in a relatively dilated state, while the nasal iris constricts in response to light.

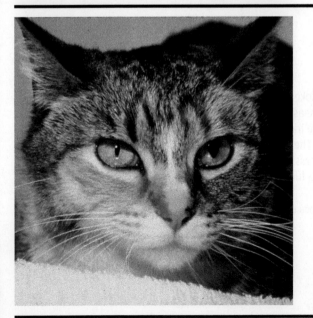

Figure 170
Spastic pupil syndrome
(4-year-old domestic shorthair)

Over the past 6 months, this cat had experienced fluctuations in pupil size and symmetry. On this particular occasion, the right pupil is miotic when compared with the left, but both retained normal pupillary light responses. Anisocoria persisted and neither pupil dilated fully in dim light. No other ocular abnormalities were present. The cat tested positive for FeLV.

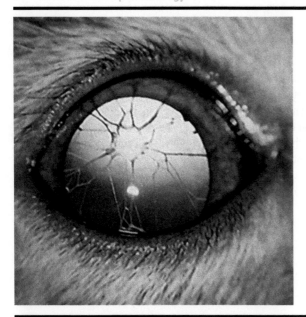

Figure 171
Persistent pupillary membranes
(6-week-old domestic shorthair)

Prior to inclusion in a nutritional study, this kitten was presented for routine ophthalmic evaluation. A network of fine pigmented strands originates from the anterior iris surface and spans the pupil. The left eye was similarly affected, as were several siblings. Vision was normal.

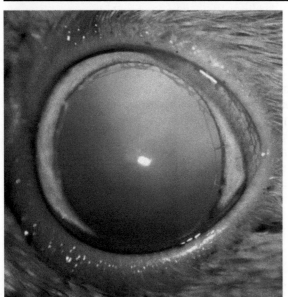

Figure 172
Persistent pupillary membranes
(8-month-old Himalayan)

This cat was presented for evaluation of bilateral conjunctivitis, accompanied by periocular discharge and marginal hyperemia. Bilateral persistent pupillary membranes (PPMs) were noted coincidentally. With the pupil pharmacologically dilated, fine strands can be seen forming a complete collarette just within the pupillary margin. Lack of pigment within the subalbinotic fundus contributes to the red reflection.

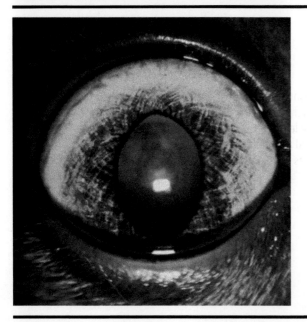

Figure 173
Chediak-Higashi syndrome
(4-year-old Persian)

The pale blue smoke color of this cat's haircoat is typical of the color dilution seen with this disease. The pale yellow iris with the basket weave appearance of the iris stroma is another characteristic of Chediak-Higashi syndrome (CHS). The nuclear and cortical lens opacities are believed to be inherited by a recessive gene other than that responsible for CHS. Figure 367 is typical of a CHS fundus.

(Image courtesy of Linda L. Collier, DVM, PhD, DACVO.)

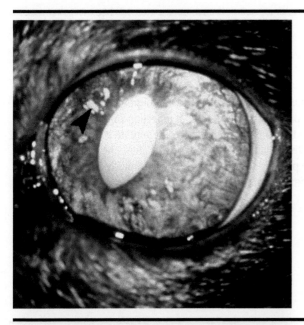

Figure 174
Iris atrophy
(18-year-old Siamese)

The tapetal reflection can easily be seen through the thinned iris. In several areas (*arrow*), the iris stroma is totally absent. The changes were bilateral but had negligible effect on the degree of pupillary excursion or pupillary light response.

(Reproduced from *Veterinary Ocular Pathology: A Comparative Review*. Dubielzig, Ketring, McLellan, Albert. Elsevier Limited, 2010.)

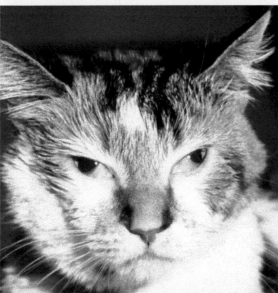

Figure 175
Feline dysautonomia
(2.5-year-old domestic shorthair)

Two weeks after arriving in the United States from Ireland, this cat became progressively anorectic and depressed, with clinical signs of weight loss, constipation, and intermittent regurgitation. Both nictitating membranes are prominent. Pupils are dilated and nonresponsive, but the cat can see. Schirmer tear test values were 0–1 mm/min. The oral and nasal mucous membranes were also dry. Megaesophagus, a distended urinary bladder and colonic distention were detected radiographically. Pharmacologic testing confirmed the autonomic dysfunction.

(Image courtesy of David D. Canton, DVM, DACVO.)

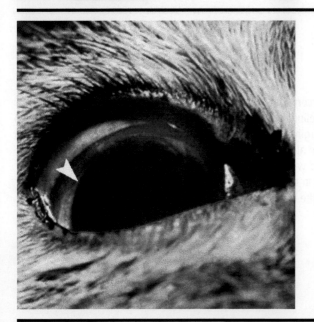

Figure 176
Feline dysautonomia
(3-year-old domestic shorthair)

Vomiting, anorexia, and listlessness developed acutely in this previously healthy animal. The pupils are widely dilated (*arrow*), but vision remained functional. Ophthalmic examination also revealed bilateral blepharospasm and Schirmer tear test values of zero. The diagnosis of dysautonomia was based on clinical signs and radiographic confirmation of megaesophagus. A tenacious mucopurulent discharge was noted on follow-up examinations.

(Image courtesy of Nancy M. Bromberg, VMD, DACVO.)

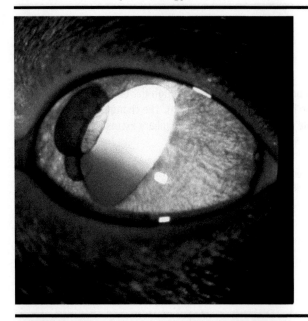

Figure 177
Iris cyst
(9.5-year-old Siamese)

The owners were unaware of the duration of a pigmented mass that originated at the pupil margin. The tapetal reflection can be seen through the lightly pigmented oval cyst, helping to differentiate it from a solid tumor. A smaller cyst is visible inferiorly. These cysts originate from the pigmented epithelium of the posterior iris surface. They are clinically benign, with no associated inflammation or vision loss.

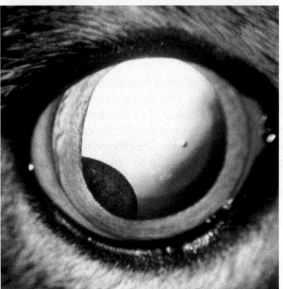

Figure 178
Iris cyst
(8-year-old domestic shorthair)

Approximately 50% of this large cyst can be seen extending beyond the pharmacologically dilated pupillary margin. The diagnosis is based on the ability to visualize the tapetal reflection through the fluid-filled cyst. Feline cysts are more likely to remain attached rather than floating freely in the anterior chamber.

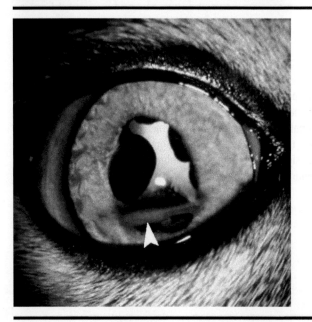

Figure 179
Iris cysts—Post-inflammatory
(2.5-year-old domestic shorthair)

A linear, dense corneal scar is visible at the arrow. The iris adheres to the corneal endothelium at both ends of the scar. A large dark mass can be seen at the pupil margin, extending onto the anterior lens surface. Several smaller masses are seen along the opposite pupillary margin. These cysts transilluminated with a bright focal light beam, although that characteristic is not apparent in the photo. The more heavily pigmented cysts may originate from the ciliary body epithelium.

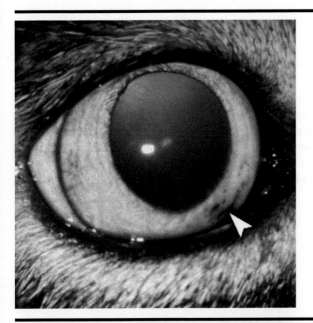

Figure 180
Anterior uveitis/Feline leukemia complex
(10.5-year-old domestic shorthair)

The owners observed bilateral squinting and ocular discharge prior to examination. A small blood-tinged fibrin clot is visible (*arrow*) in the ventronasal anterior chamber. Temporal iris vessels are congested. Aqueous flare and keratic precipitates contribute to the haze seen through the dilated pupil. The fundus is depicted in Figure 298. The only positive serologic test was that for FeLV.

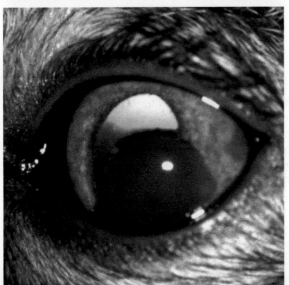

Figure 181
Anterior uveitis/Feline leukemia complex
(8-month-old domestic shorthair)

This cat had a 4-day history of anorexia, lethargy, and bilateral ocular pain indicated by squinting. A large blood-tinged fibrin clot is present in the anterior chamber of the left eye. The entire iris face appears reddened because of dilation of surface vessels. The posterior segment was normal in both eyes. A test for FeLV was positive.

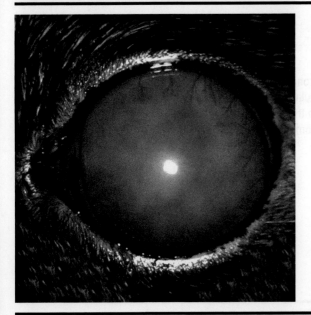

Figure 182
Anterior uveitis/Feline leukemia complex
(2-year-old domestic shorthair)

The owners were unaware of any ocular disease in this outdoor cat until he was observed bumping into objects. Both eyes were similarly affected. The cornea is severely edematous and superficially vascularized 360 degrees. The pupil is miotic and difficult to visualize, but the anterior chamber is shallow because of iris swelling. The posterior segment could not be observed in either eye. The only positive serologic test was for feline leukemia virus.

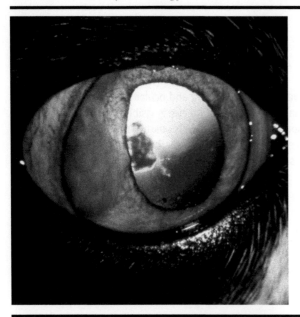

Figure 183
Anterior uveitis/Feline leukemia complex
(14-year-old domestic shorthair)

The referring veterinarian reported a positive FeLV test on this cat, presented with a 2-day history of a cloudy right eye. This right pupil has been pharmacologically dilated but response is incomplete. The temporal iris is focally thickened and hyperemic. Mild aqueous flare and deposits of pigment and inflammatory cells on the anterior lens capsule indicate breakdown of the blood-aqueous barrier. The left eye and posterior segments of both eyes were normal.

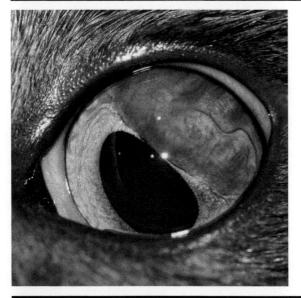

Figure 184
Iris abscess
(8-month-old domestic shorthair)

This young cat was presented with a 3-week history of an enlarging mass affecting the temporal iris. There were no additional ocular abnormalities in either eye. All serologies for FeLV, FIV, toxoplasmosis, and *Bartonella* were negative. An ocular ultrasound confirmed that the mass was limited to the iris. A fine-needle aspirate consisted of small lymphocytes, PMNs, and histocytic cells. No neoplastic cells were identified. With a combination of oral and topical antibiotics and prednisolone, the hyperemia and swelling decreased. The kitten has now been controlled with topical antibiotics/dexamethasone for approximately 7 months. The smooth elevated mass is more vascular and pigment migration at the pupil margin is negligible in comparison to cases of iris neoplasia.

(Image courtesy of Noelle La Croix, DVM, DACVO.)

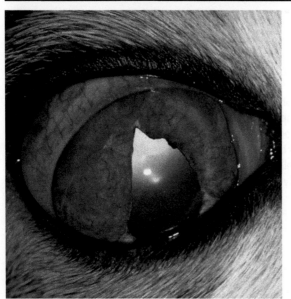

Figure 185
Lymphoma
(15-year-old domestic shorthair)

Duration of this condition was unknown. The iris is diffusely swollen, prominently vascularized, and darker in color than the normal left eye. The dyscoria is due to the neoplastic infiltrate within the iris stroma. Histopathology confirmed the diagnosis of lymphoma.

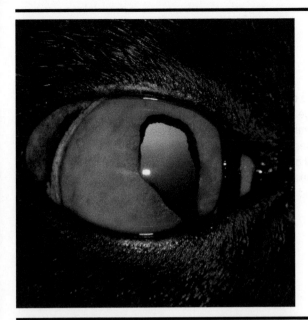

Figure 186
Lymphoma
(7-year-old domestic shorthair)

The owner noticed a progressive change in the right eye over the past 4 months. An isolated lesion in the left eye had gone undetected. The pink to flesh-colored thickening, most obvious in the temporal iris, is typical of this neoplasia. The pigmented swelling at the pupil margin and the misshapen pupil are also common findings. The cat had a faint aqueous flare but showed no subjective signs of pain.

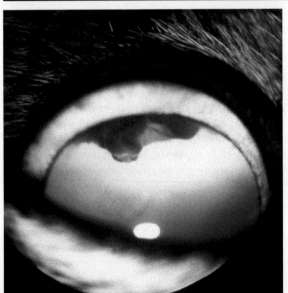

Figure 187
Lymphoma
(4-year-old domestic shorthair)

This cat was initially presented for evaluation of a mass in the opposite eye. An irregular, darkly colored, vascularized mass protrudes into the posterior chamber. The mass could be seen only after the pupil was dilated. There was no evidence of active inflammation or posterior segment disease in either eye. A FeLV test was negative. The bilateral masses were diagnosed as lymphoma on the basis of histopathologic examination.

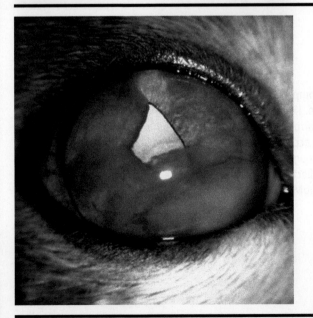

Figure 188
Lymphoma/Anterior uveitis
(7-year-old domestic shorthair)

An intraocular mass had been noticed by the owner 1 week prior to examination. A large pale fibrin clot is present in the ventral aspect of the anterior chamber. The pupil shape is distorted by a swollen, prominently vascularized iris and the presence of posterior synechia. The iris swelling also compromises the anterior chamber depth. Intraocular pressure is elevated. No abnormalities were identified in the opposite eye or within the posterior segment of this eye. A feline leukemia virus test was positive. Ocular lymphoma was diagnosed on histopathology.

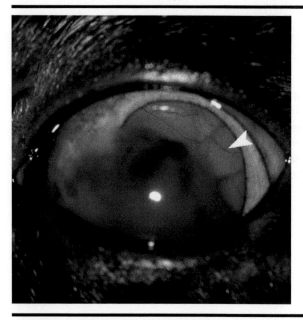

Figure 189
Lymphoma
(7-year-old domestic shorthair)

The owners noticed cloudiness of the eye beginning 1 month prior to this photograph. A large fibrinous clot with areas of hemorrhage fills two-thirds of the anterior chamber, obscuring most of the swollen and vascularized nasal iris. Retinal vessels (*arrow*) can be seen through the dilated and unresponsive pupil owing to a complete retinal detachment. Histopathological examination found neoplastic lymphocytes within the ciliary body, choroid and optic nerve.

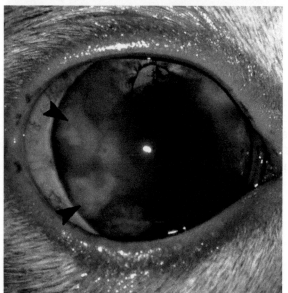

Figure 190
Anterior uveitis/Feline leukemia complex/Feline immunodeficiency virus
(11-year-old domestic shorthair)

This cat had a history of a red eye for 1 week. The anterior chamber contains a large fibrinohemorrhagic clot. The iris vessels are dilated and a white, fluffy mass occupies the temporal chamber (*arrows*). The pupil is largely obscured but is misshapen because of posterior synechia. The posterior segment could not be visualized. Intraocular pressure was elevated. Tests for FeLV and FIV were both positive.

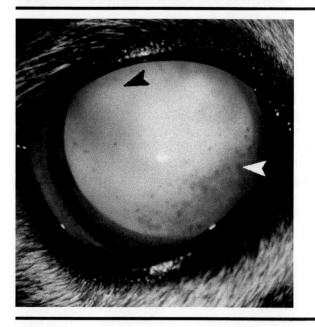

Figure 191
Anterior uveitis/Pars planitis/Feline immunodeficiency virus
(6-year-old domestic shorthair)

The presenting complaint mentioned cloudy eyes and decreasing vision of 2 weeks' duration. Keratic precipitates are prominent in the nasal corneal quadrant (*white arrow*). Inflammatory cells originating from the inflamed ciliary body have accumulated within the anterior vitreous, creating the opacity noted through the pupil (*black arrow*). These cells also diminish the overall tapetal reflection. Serology was positive for FIV but negative for FeLV and Toxoplasma IgM.

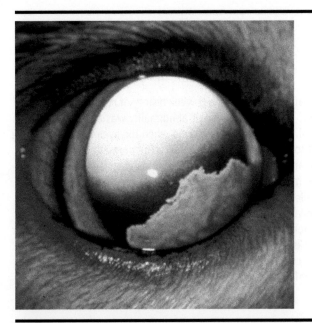

Figure 192
Anterior uveitis/Feline infectious peritonitis
(1.5-year-old domestic shorthair)

This cat was presented with a 2-day history of a cloudy eye. A large white fibrin clot is visible in the ventral anterior chamber. Mild aqueous flare was present in both eyes, as were focal retinal exudates and perivascular cuffing. Repeated tests for FeLV and toxoplasmosis were negative. The total serum protein was 8.1 g/dl. A presumptive diagnosis of FIP was made on the basis of ocular signs and laboratory findings.

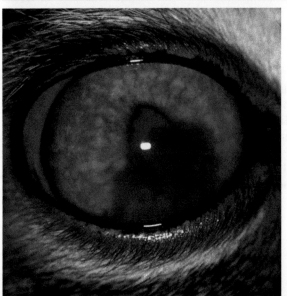

Figure 193
Anterior uveitis/Feline infectious peritonitis
(7-year-old domestic shorthair)

Anorexia and weight loss had been observed for several weeks. Redness of the eye was noted 3 days prior to this photograph. Aqueous flare is present in this and the opposite eye. A blood-tinged fibrin clot within the anterior chamber contains spots of pigment. The iris appears orange in color because of its vascular congestion. Posterior synechiae are present, with pigment deposits on the anterior lens capsule. The posterior segment is poorly visualized in this eye, but the opposite fundus is shown in Figure 303.

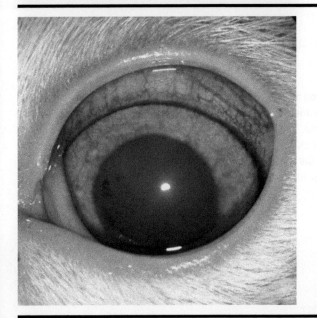

Figure 194
Anterior uveitis/Feline infectious peritonitis
(3-year-old domestic shorthair)

Initial lesions developed in this left eye. One month later, uveitis also developed in the right eye. Dilation of conjunctival and episcleral vessels contribute to the hyperemia. Aqueous flare mutes the iris detail, with diffuse rubeosis iridis and blood-tinged keratic precipitates at the 9-o'clock position. The red reflex noted through the pupil is caused by massive posterior segment hemorrhage. A total protein of 10.6 g/dl and globulin of 7.4 g/dl were the only notable laboratory findings. Serology failed to identify an infectious cause. At necropsy, ocular lesions and general pathological findings were compatible with FIP.

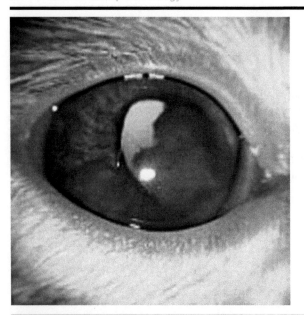

Figure 195
Anterior uveitis/Feline infectious peritonitis
(6-month-old domestic shorthair)

This adolescent cat presented with a 6-week history of red, cloudy eyes, and intermittent fever. The only hematologic abnormality was an elevated serum protein of 8.4 g/dl. The patient was referred when the eyes failed to improve despite frequent topical corticosteroid therapy. The normally blue iris is discolored by inflammatory cells and prominent iris vessels. A large fibrin clot obscures the medial pupil. Fibrin and cells also obscure the iris surface temporally. Detailed fundus evaluation was hindered both by resistance to pharmacologic dilation and by the anterior chamber debris, but dazzle reflex and menace response were present. The left eye was similarly affected. Over the next few weeks, the anterior chamber exudates increased, completely and permanently covering the pupils and leaving the patient functionally blind. FIP was confirmed on necropsy 4 months after this initial visit.

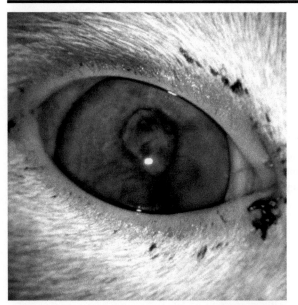

Figure 196
Anterior uveitis/Feline infectious peritonitis
(5-year-old domestic shorthair)

This cat was functionally blind due to severe anterior segment inflammation in this right eye and diffuse posterior segment involvement in the left eye (see Figure 308). The mild corneal edema and a fibrinohemorrhagic exudate in the anterior chamber prevent clear visualization of the swollen hemorrhagic iris. Posterior synechia have altered the pupillary shape. The total protein was 10.8 g/dl, globulin was 8.8 g/dl, and the cat had a profound lymphopenia.

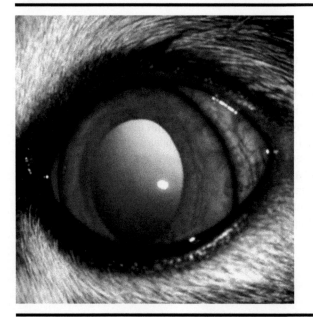

Figure 197
Anterior uveitis/Toxoplasmosis
(6-month-old domestic shorthair)

This cat had been squinting the left eye for 1 month. On examination, blepharospasm and mild conjunctival hyperemia are seen, along with subtle perilimbal edema. The hazy appearance through the dilated pupil is due to moderate aqueous flare. The iris is diffusely swollen. The posterior segment of this eye and the entire right eye were normal. A FeLV test was negative, but the IgM titer for *Toxoplasma gondii* was positive at 1:128.

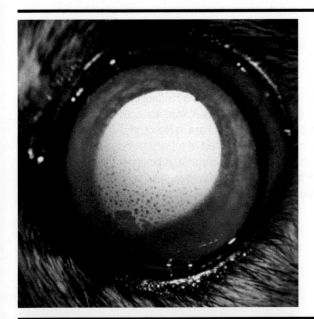

Figure 198
Anterior uveitis/Toxoplasmosis
(8-year-old domestic shorthair)

The history was vague in this outdoor cat. Both eyes were similarly affected. Many variably sized keratic precipitates can be seen scattered on the inferior corneal endothelial surface. A moderate aqueous flare is present. The iris is swollen and iridal vessels are dilated temporally. Retinitis was present in both eyes. A FeLV test was negative; the *Toxoplasma gondii* titer was positive at greater than 1:400. Toxoplasmosis was the presumptive etiology based on the clinical signs and laboratory tests.

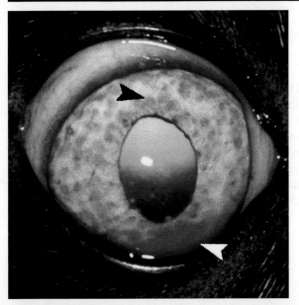

Figure 199
Anterior uveitis/Toxoplasmosis
(4.5-year-old domestic shorthair)

For several weeks, the owner had noticed her cat squinting. Keratic precipitates and a large fibrin clot (*white arrow*) can be seen in the ventral anterior chamber. Mild aqueous flare is present, along with mild vascularization of the iris face. Small off-white circular swellings scattered across the iris face are referred to as Busacca nodules (*black arrow*) and are the result of focal accumulations of inflammatory cells. Posterior segment findings were limited to a mild hyalitis. FeLV and FIV tests were negative. One month later, the initial Toxoplasma IgM titer of 1:128 rose to 1:16,384.

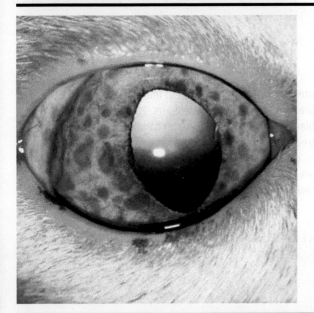

Figure 200
Anterior uveitis/Toxoplasmosis
(6-year-old domestic shorthair)

This indoor/outdoor cat had been squinting its right eye. The most striking ocular finding consists of multiple dark gray inflammatory nodules dotting the iris surface. Vessels can be easily seen across the temporal iris face. A mild aqueous flare was also present. The left eye was completely normal as was the posterior segment of this eye. The presumptive diagnosis was based on an IgM titer of 1:40 and an IgG titer of 1:2048 for *Toxoplasma gondii*.

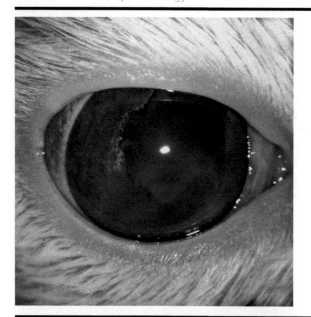

Figure 201
Anterior uveitis/Toxoplasmosis
(11-year-old domestic shorthair)

Recently lethargic, this cat presented with a reddened right eye of 1 week's duration. The conjunctiva is notably hyperemic. Aqueous flare is present but fibrin is responsible for the ill-defined haze in the ventral anterior chamber. The intensely hyperemic iris is a product of rubeosis iridis, a fine network of new vessels branching across the iris surface. A posterior synechia alters the temporal pupillary margin. The posterior segment could not be visualized. No lesions were found in the left eye. The only positive serology was a 1:400 Toxoplasma titer.

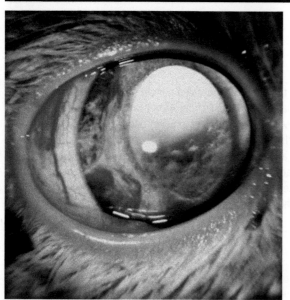

Figure 202
Anterior uveitis/Toxoplasmosis/Histoplasmosis
(6-month-old Persian)

A veterinarian had treated this cat's bilateral anterior uveitis for 10 days before referral. Both eyes were similarly affected. A white flocculent material composed of fibrin and inflammatory cells spans the ventral pupillary space. The base of the temporal iris is effaced by prominently vascularized nodules. Focal retinal edema was seen in both eyes; a bullous retinal detachment was present in the left eye. *Toxoplasma gondii* titers were positive (IgM 1:1024; IgG 1:256). The cat developed pneumonia and was euthanatized. *Histoplasma capsulatum* was identified in the lung, liver, spleen, kidney, and iris.

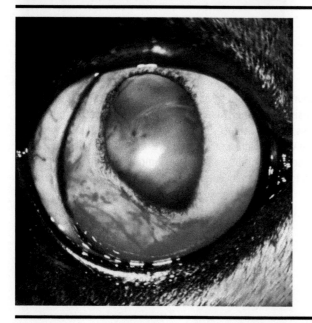

Figure 203
Anterior uveitis/Histoplasmosis
(3-year-old domestic shorthair)

The pupil is distorted by a vascularized mass in the ventrotemporal iris. Vessels are also prominent in other iris quadrants. The ventral shadow is produced by cellular debris within the anterior chamber. Inflammatory cells in the anterior vitreous give the pupil a cloudy appearance and should be differentiated from cataract and retinal detachment. A diagnosis of histoplasmosis was confirmed on bone marrow aspirate. Ocular signs improved with therapy, but the cat was euthanatized because of systemic complications.

(Image courtesy of Art J. Quinn, DVM, DACVO.)

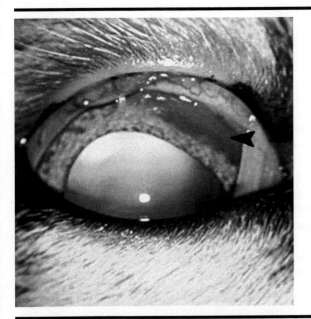

Figure 204
Anterior uveitis/Histoplasmosis
(8-year-old domestic shorthair)

This farm cat was presented when the owners noted several skin lesions along with squinting of both eyes. The conjunctiva is chemotic and hyperemic. The dark area at the limbus (*arrow*) is due to corneal edema and vascularization of the underlying iris. Mild aqueous flare is present. The pupil has been dilated to examine the fundus (see Figure 312). The left eye was similarly affected, but also had a large lid granuloma (see Figure 68). *Histoplasma capsulatum* organisms were recovered from the skin lesions, oral ulcers, and the eye. Serology was positive for FeLV but negative for histoplasmosis.

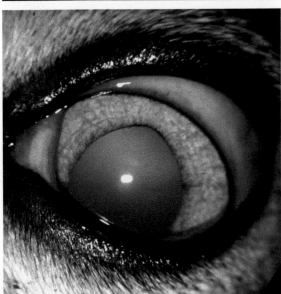

Figure 205
Anterior uveitis/Histoplasmosis
(2-year-old domestic shorthair)

At presentation, this cat had a 5-month history of carpal pain and lameness and had now been blind for 4 weeks. The left eye demonstrates faint aqueous flare, a moderately dilated, nonresponsive pupil, and subtle leukocoria associated with severe retinal disease. Anterior uveitis and a diffuse cataract prevented posterior segment examination of the opposite eye. Serologic tests were negative for common mycoses, toxoplasmosis, FIV, FeLV, and *Bartonella*. Histopathologically, lesions in the right eye were characterized as idiopathic lymphogranulomatous panuveitis with retinitis. No etiologic agents were identified. Progression of the uveitis can be seen in Figure 206.

(Reproduced from *Veterinary Ocular Pathology: A Comparative Review*. Dubielzig, Ketring, McLellan, Albert. Elsevier Limited, 2010.)

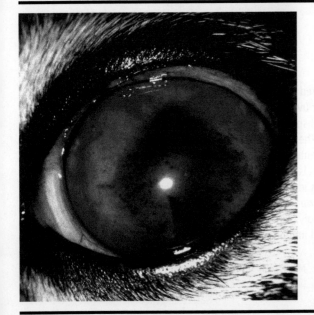

Figure 206
Anterior uveitis/Histoplasmosis
(2-year-old domestic shorthair)

This is the same eye as that depicted in Figure 205 approximately 6 weeks later. The iris is severely swollen with posterior synechia that limit pupillary size and distort its shape. The intense red color is attributed to free blood that coats the corneal endothelium and iris. In light of the severe hemorrhagic anterior uveitis, this eye was also enucleated. Histopathology results were similar to findings in the right eye, with no apparent etiology. Two months later, a fine-needle aspirate of a swollen submandibular lymph node yielded yeast-like organisms within macrophages compatible with *Histoplasma capsulatum*. This case is compatible with Presumed Ocular Histoplasmosis Syndrome (POHS) reported in man.

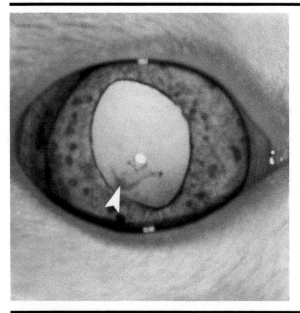

Figure 207
Anterior uveitis/Cryptococcosis
(11-year-old domestic shorthair)

Primary complaints in this case included an enlarged right eye and a tendency to circle to the right. The globe was slightly enlarged in association with a mild intraocular pressure elevation. Faint aqueous flare is present. A fibrin clot is seen (*arrow*) on the lens surface. Many dark focal inflammatory nodules are present on the iris surface. The tapetal reflection and retinal detail are decreased by inflammatory cells within the anterior vitreous. Focal retinal edema was present along the retinal vessels of the opposite eye (see Figure 314). Serology for FeLV, FIV, and toxoplasmosis were negative. The titer for *Cryptococcus* spp antigen was positive at 1:1024.

(Reproduced from *Veterinary Ocular Pathology: A Comparative Review*. Dubielzig, Ketring, McLellan, Albert. Elsevier Limited, 2010.)

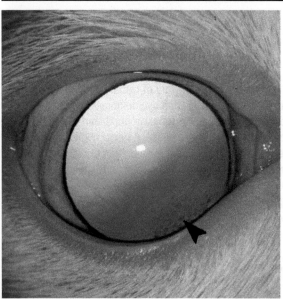

Figure 208
Anterior uveitis/Cryptococcosis
(5-year-old domestic shorthair)

Squinting called attention to this cat's bilateral corneal cloudiness. The normally blue iris is gray in color and mildly swollen. A faint aqueous flare accompanies keratic precipitates seen inferiorly (*arrow*). Bilateral chorioretinitis was also present (see Figure 317). The only positive serology was a 1:1024 titer for *Cryptococcus neoformans* antigen.

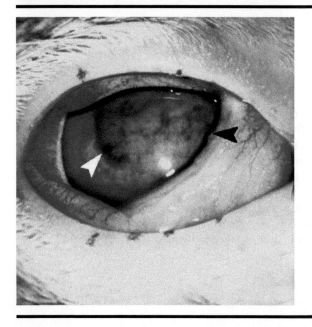

Figure 209
Anterior uveitis/Blastomycosis
(8-year-old domestic shorthair)

The cat was referred when he failed to respond to therapy for severe unilateral anterior uveitis and secondary glaucoma. The right nictitans protrudes as a nonspecific sign of ocular pain; its free margin is identified by the *black arrow*. The conjunctiva is edematous and severely hyperemic. Fibrin within the anterior chamber (*white arrow*) obscures the pupil. Temporal iris vessels are prominent. The opposite eye was normal. A thoracic mass was identified radiographically. Blastomycosis was diagnosed when organisms were identified cytologically within a skin nodule on the muzzle. Interestingly, serology for *Blastomyces dermatitidis* was negative using the agar-gel immunodiffusion method.

(Image courtesy of Paul Miller, DVM, DACVO.)

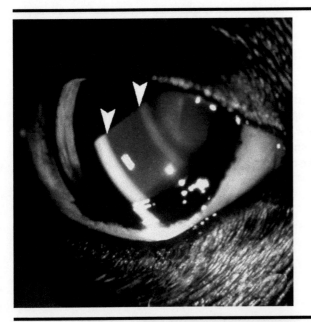

Figure 210
Anterior uveitis/Blastomycosis
(10-year-old domestic shorthair)

Toxoplasma-associated anterior uveitis had been diagnosed on the basis of positive serology, but the cat was referred when no improvement was seen following appropriate therapy. Lesions were confined to the right eye. The anterior chamber (between the *white arrows*) appears cloudy in the slit lamp image because of an increase in aqueous protein, i.e., flare. A retinal detachment was also present in this eye. Blastomycosis was diagnosed when organisms were identified in a subretinal aspirate.

(Image courtesy of Paul Miller, DVM, DACVO.)

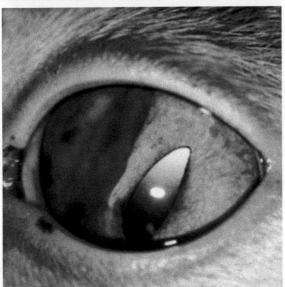

Figure 211
Anterior uveitis/Coccidioidomycosis
(2-year-old domestic shorthair)

Referred for evaluation of a presumed iris tumor, this cat also had a nail bed infection affecting one paw. Ocular lesions were unilateral and restricted to the anterior segment of the left eye. A large vascularized mass effaces the medial aspect of the iris. Mild aqueous flare and scattered areas of iris vascularization are also present. Histopathology of the globe and nail identified *Coccidioides immitis* spherules within areas of pyogranulomatous inflammation.

(Image courtesy of Paul M. Barrett, DVM, DACVO.)

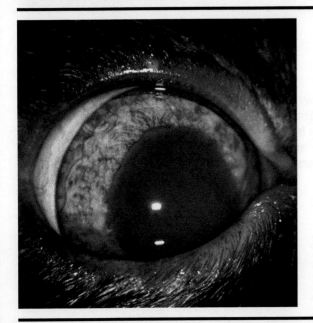

Figure 212
Anterior uveitis/Polymicrobial etiology
(11-year-old Himalayan)

This patient arrived with a history of weight loss, coupled with the onset of anterior uveitis 4 days beforehand. Severe rubeosis iridis is present, altering the color of the normally blue iris. A large hemorrhagic clot completely occludes the pupil. Pharmacologic dilation afforded a limited view of the posterior segment, where severe chorioretinitis obscured fundus detail. The left eye was normal. Tests for FeLV, FIV, and all common mycoses were negative. Serology for *Bartonella* spp was positive, as was an IgM/IgG titer for toxoplasmosis at 1:1024. Histopathology of the enucleated eye revealed a multifocal lymphoplasmacytic and pyogranulomatous uveitis and retinitis, with yeast-like organisms consistent with *Histoplasma capsulatum*. All three infectious agents were targeted therapeutically. Two months after initial examination, the cat developed mild anterior uveitis in the left eye. Fungal serology remained negative. The post-treatment *Toxoplasma* titer decreased to 1:256 while the *Bartonella* titer decreased fourfold.

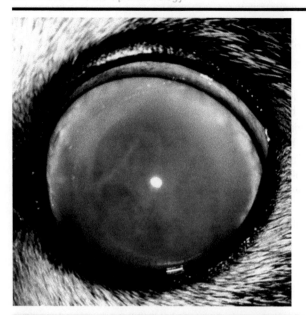

Figure 213
Anterior uveitis/Bartonellosis
(15-year-old domestic shorthair)

The owner noticed the cat squinting both eyes for 2 days prior to examination. Ocular lesions were similar bilaterally. A large gray fibrinous clot in the anterior chamber obscures iris and pupillary detail. Although difficult to view, the posterior segment appeared normal. *Bartonella henselae* was the only infectious agent implicated serologically.

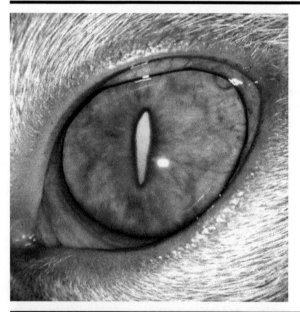

Figure 214
Anterior uveitis/Bartonellosis
(6-month-old Siamese)

Bartonella spp had been serologically implicated in a previous episode of unilateral anterior uveitis and pinnae dermatitis in this kitten. The skin lesions were compatible with bacillary angiomatosis due to Bartonellosis described in humans. This photograph of the once normal left eye was taken 1 month after the initial diagnosis, 2 weeks after the termination of a 10-day treatment regimen, and 24 hours following onchyectomy and ovariohysterectomy. The normally blue iris is swollen and flesh-colored. Moderate aqueous flare accompanies severe iris vessel engorgement and a miotic pupil. The previously inflamed right eye and pinnae were normal on this day. All evidence of anterior uveitis resolved within 5 days, using only an oral antibiotic selected for its efficacy against *Bartonella* spp.

(Reproduced from *Veterinary Ocular Pathology: A Comparative Review*. Dubielzig, Ketring, McLellan, Albert. Elsevier Limited, 2010.)

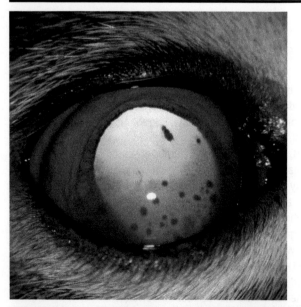

Figure 215
Anterior uveitis/Bartonellosis
(7-month-old domestic shorthair)

Lethargy and fever preceded the onset of bilateral blepharospasm in this young adult patient. Clinical findings were similar in both eyes. There is a diffusely swollen iris, moderate aqueous flare, and numerous keratic precipitates, the larger of which appear dark against the tapetal reflection. Of all serology submitted, only that for *Bartonella henselae* was positive.

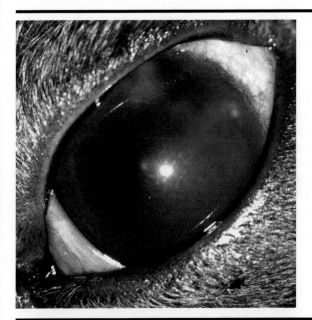

Figure 216
Anterior uveitis/Bartonellosis
(1-year-old domestic shorthair)

The owner felt this bilateral condition had progressed quickly over the last 5 days. Diffusely dispersed red blood cells within the anterior chamber obscure intraocular detail. The pupil was miotic at presentation but dilated in response to medication. The only significant laboratory finding was a positive serologic test for *Bartonella henselae*.

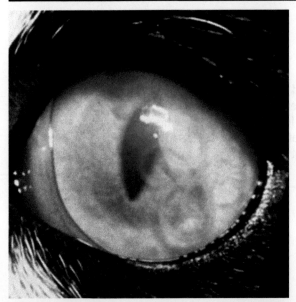

Figure 217
Anterior uveitis/Dirofilariasis
(2.5-year-old domestic shorthair)

A viable immature adult *Dirofilaria immitis* can be seen in the temporal anterior chamber. Mild corneal edema is present, a sign attributed to altered endothelial function. The parasite's role includes both physical damage to the endothelium as well as toxic effects of its metabolic by-products.

(Image courtesy of Ben W. Johnson, DVM, DACVO.)

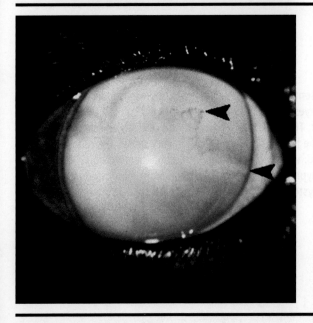

Figure 218
Anterior uveitis/Myiasis
(1-year-old domestic shorthair)

A cloudy eye was noted in conjunction with the acute of tetraparesis. Subconjunctival hemorrhage accounts for the intense red coloration of the temporal conjunctiva. The cornea is diffusely edematous, almost obscuring an intraocular *Cuterebra* larva (*arrows*). Anterior chamber detail is further obscured by fibrin and cellular debris. The parasite was identified following its surgical removal from the anterior chamber.

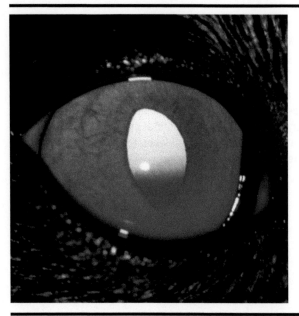

Figure 219
Anterior uveitis/Lipid flare
(9-month-old domestic shorthair)

Presented due to the rapid onset of cloudy eyes, this cat was diagnosed with a mild, bilateral anterior uveitis. A gray haze obscures iris detail, especially in the ventral half of the anterior chamber. The opacity is the result of lipid-laden aqueous, not corneal edema. Lipemia retinalis was also present bilaterally, similar to that in Figure 368. The cat was diagnosed with diabetes mellitus, with an initial blood glucose of 460 mg/dl. The cause of the anterior uveitis was not determined.

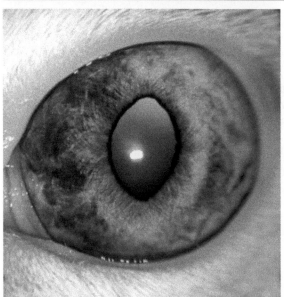

Figure 220
Anterior uveitis/Systemic hypertension
(16.5-year-old domestic shorthair)

Owners noticed red spots recently developing in the left eye. The cat had a history of chronic renal disease but no previous ocular problems. Multiple, poorly defined red foci in the medial iris are the result of hemorrhage within the iris stroma. A lateral bullous retinal detachment was also present in the same eye. The right eye was normal. The mean systolic blood pressure was 220 mm Hg.

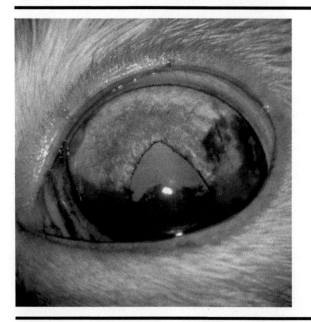

Figure 221
Anterior uveitis/Systemic hypertension
(14-year-old domestic shorthair)

This cat was presented with acute complaints of decreased vision and redness in both eyes. Hyphema creates the dark red color within the ventral anterior chamber. The outline of a darker blood clot can be seen just emerging from the hemorrhage over the pupillary space. The retina was partially detached, with subretinal and intraretinal hemorrhage. The right eye had a total hyphema preventing visualization of the posterior segment. The cat's mean systolic blood pressure was greater than 300 mm Hg.

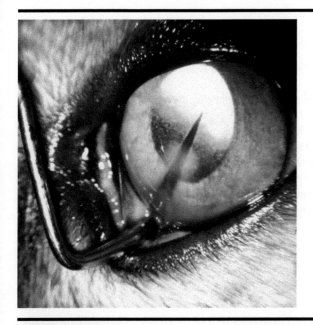

Figure 222
Anterior uveitis/Foreign body
(2-year-old domestic shorthair)

Several hours after acute onset of ocular pain, this cat was presented for evaluation. A large thorn has penetrated the cornea at the limbus and has also impaled the lens. Corneal edema is present, along with aqueous flare. The iris is swollen and severely hyperemic. This type of lens damage may set the stage for a future post-traumatic sarcoma.

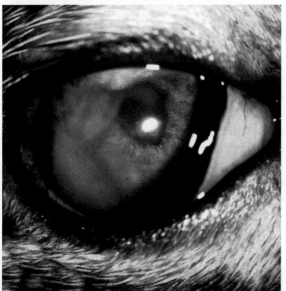

Figure 223
Anterior uveitis/Trauma
(1-year-old domestic shorthair)

This kitten was notorious for playing with sewing needles and was presented for evaluation of an acutely painful, red and cloudy right eye. The temporal cornea is opaque due to severe edema and deep vascularization. Moderate aqueous flare and fibrin can be seen in the anterior chamber, the latter extending from the temporal pupil margin to the area of edema. Posterior synechia contribute to the small irregular pupil. Severe iritis with neovascularization of the iris surface is most notable temporally. A diffusely opaque lens obscured posterior segment detail. Skull radiographs identified a needle within the orbit. The needle was found lodged in the inferior temporal globe during enucleation.

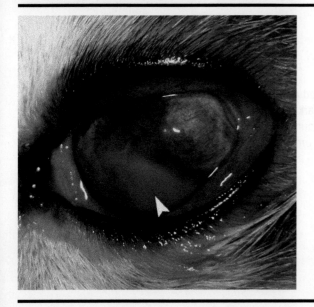

Figure 224
Septic lens implantation
(13-year-old domestic shorthair)

This cat was seen 1 year ago with a full-thickness corneal scar, an incipient cataract and a mild uveitis, all attributed to a suspected penetrating injury. Now there is marked conjunctival inflammation surrounding a buphthalmic globe. Iris bombé is easily recognized temporally, where the green iris balloons into the anterior chamber. Hypopyon (*arrow*) and a reddish brown fibrinous sheet occlude the pupil. IOP was elevated to 43 mm Hg. Histopathologically, gram-positive cocci were found within the lens, accompanied by severe neutrophilic, lymphocytic and plasmacytic infiltrates throughout the globe.

(Image courtesy of Jean Stiles, DVM, MS, DACVO.)

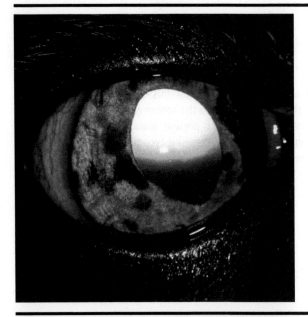

Figure 225
Neoplasia/Feline diffuse iris melanoma
(9-year-old domestic shorthair)

The owners noticed progressive darkening of the iris, but comfort and vision remained unchanged. Multiple flat, pigmented foci are randomly scattered across the iris face. No exfoliated pigment cells were seen within the aqueous or deposited onto the anterior lens capsule. Progression of the pigmentation is illustrated in Figure 226.

(Reproduced from *Veterinary Ocular Pathology: A Comparative Review*. Dubielzig, Ketring, McLellan, Albert. Elsevier Limited, 2010.)

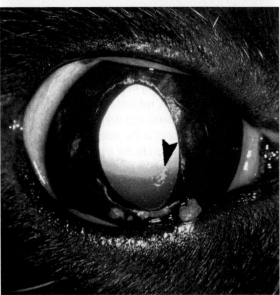

Figure 226
Neoplasia/Feline diffuse iris melanoma
(12.5-year-old domestic shorthair)

This is the same eye as that in Figure 225, examined 3.5 years later. The iris is now diffusely pigmented. Iris thickening is also present in some areas, although the change is not easily appreciated in the figure. Exfoliated cells are present on the anterior lens capsule (*arrow*). An unrelated papillomatous mass is seen on the lower lid margin.

(Reproduced from *Veterinary Ocular Pathology: A Comparative Review*. Dubielzig, Ketring, McLellan, Albert. Elsevier Limited, 2010.)

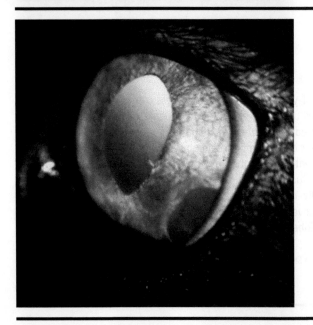

Figure 227
Neoplasia/Amelanotic melanoma
(4-year-old domestic shorthair)

The owners noticed a red spot in the eye 10 days prior to this photograph. A well-delineated dark red mass can be seen at the base of the iris. Mild aqueous flare accounts for the hazy tapetal reflection. Histopathologic diagnosis was an amelanotic melanoma.

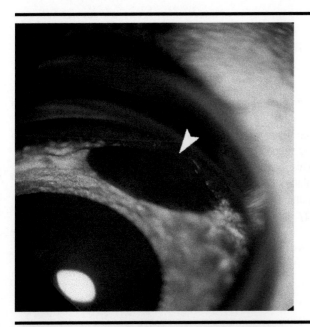

Figure 228
Neoplasia/Melanoma
(1.5-year-old domestic shorthair)

The owner noticed a dark spot in the eye that had gradually increased in size over the past 6 months. This gonioscopic view shows a well-defined pigmented mass that rises slightly above the surrounding iris. The pigmented tissue extends into the drainage angle and onto the pectinate ligaments (*arrow*).

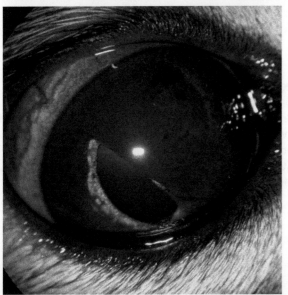

Figure 229
Neoplasia/Feline diffuse iris melanoma
(9-year-old domestic shorthair)

The owner was unaware of the duration of a color change in the right eye. A heavily pigmented mass fills two-thirds of the anterior chamber and extends into the temporal iridocorneal angle. Only a small area of yellow iris remains along the temporal pupillary margin. The mass could also be seen extending into the posterior chamber and infiltrating the nasal ciliary processes. On histopathology, neoplastic cells were widespread in the anterior uvea while the sclera, retina, and optic nerve were largely spared.

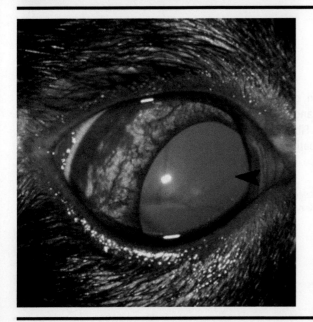

Figure 230
Neoplasia/Amelanotic melanoma
(3-year-old Siamese)

According to the owner, the cornea and iris in this cat had become vascularized over a 2-week period. The superior temporal cornea is edematous and deeply vascularized. The adjacent scleral vessels are also severely congested. The base of the temporal iris is thickened, prominently vascularized, and its background pale in comparison to the normal blue color. Retinal vessels (*arrow*) are easily seen through the pupil, an indication of a complete retinal detachment caused by subretinal fluid accumulation. Histopathologic diagnosis was iris melanoma, with extension into the ciliary body, choroid, and sclera.

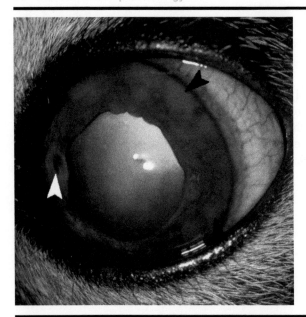

Figure 231
Neoplasia/ Feline diffuse iris melanoma
(9.5-year-old domestic shorthair)

This cat was presented with a 10-day history of squinting and redness of the left eye. The iris is diffusely discolored. Mild aqueous flare accompanies subtle stippling on the anterior lens capsule that suggests cellular debris. The pupil is irregularly shaped, with increased pigmentation along its margin. Medial iris synechia (both anterior and posterior) are indicated by the white arrow. Multifocal ill-defined cottony gray nodules are scattered throughout the iris, creating an irregular surface contour. The diagnosis was confirmed by histopathology.

(Reproduced from *Veterinary Ocular Pathology: A Comparative Review*. Dubielzig, Ketring, McLellan, Albert. Elsevier Limited, 2010.)

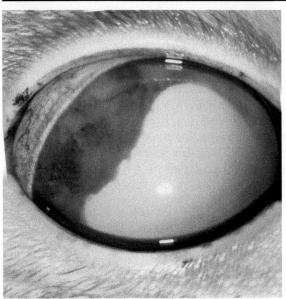

Figure 232
Neoplasia/Amelanotic melanoma
(12-year-old domestic shorthair)

The owner had been aware of the patient's squinting and cloudiness for 1 week. There is diffuse corneal edema and moderate aqueous flare, both contributing to the hazy view of an intraocular mass. The pupil is dilated and nonresponsive. A vascularized and variably colored flocculent mass can be seen in the temporal and superior iris. Intraocular pressure was elevated to 36 mm Hg. On histopathology, the mass consisted of mainly nonpigmented neoplastic cells, some of which were found in the scleral venous plexus.

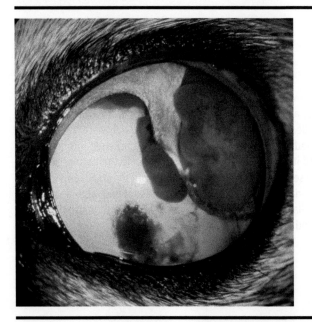

Figure 233
Neoplasia/Iridociliary adenoma
(9-year-old domestic longhair)

This vascularized, dark pink mass eroded through the iris base and adjacent drainage angle and now extends from the posterior chamber into the pupillary space. Fibrin and clotted blood are present in the ventral anterior chamber. Histopathology confirmed the diagnosis. A tumor also developed in the second eye, depicted in Figure 234.

(Reproduced from *Veterinary Ocular Pathology: A Comparative Review*. Dubielzig, Ketring, McLellan, Albert. Elsevier Limited, 2010.)

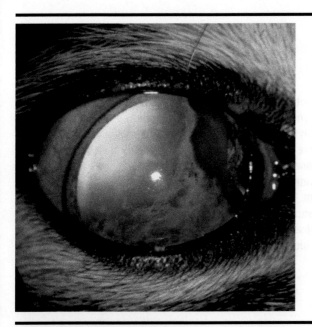

Figure 234
Neoplasia/Iridociliary adenoma
(17-year-old domestic longhair)

This is the right eye of the cat seen in Figure 233, examined 8 years later. Its left eye had been enucleated because of an extensive iridociliary adenoma. The owners noticed the cat squinting for several days prior to examination. Prior to dilation of the pupil, the only obvious abnormality was a blood-tinged fibrinous exudate in the anterior chamber. Following dilation, a dark pink, irregular mass can be seen originating from the posterior surface of the iris and the ciliary body.

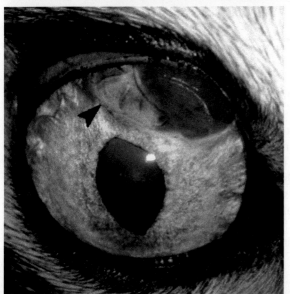

Figure 235
Neoplasia/Iridociliary adenoma
(12-year-old domestic mediumhair)

The owners only recently noticed a red color developing in their cat's iris. There were no subjective signs of pain. The cornea and aqueous humor remain clear. A dark red neoplasm penetrates the superior iris base. The adjacent 12-o'clock iris (*arrow*) is elevated and its surface architecture altered by the proliferating mass, but the tumor has not yet broken through the anterior surface in this region.

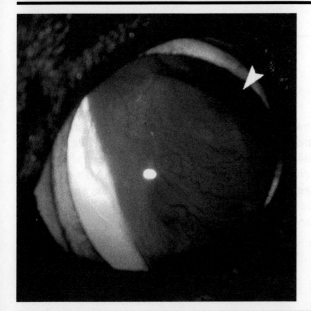

Figure 236
Neoplasia/Iridociliary adenoma
(10-year-old domestic shorthair)

This patient's pupil has been dilated for the examination. A massive well-vascularized tumor originates in the posterior chamber. Mild fibrin adjacent to the mass distorts what little can be seen of the tapetal reflection. Pigment (*arrow*) migrating from the posterior iris or ciliary body discolors the peripheral tumor surface. Surprisingly, there is minimal discomfort and only subtle uveitis associated with the tumor.

(Reproduced from *Veterinary Ocular Pathology: A Comparative Review*. Dubielzig, Ketring, McLellan, Albert. Elsevier Limited, 2010.)

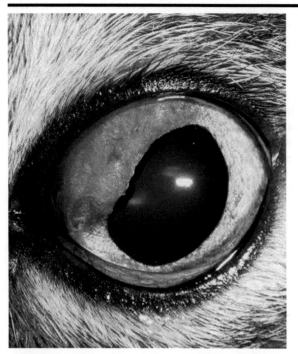

Figure 237
Neoplasia/Spindle cell tumor
(12-year-old domestic shorthair)

The owners first noted this enlarging mass 5 days prior to the photograph. A nodular nonpigmented mass in the medial iris is mildly vascularized. The adjacent pupil is dyscoric, with pigment migration and proliferation at the pupil margin. There were no other ocular abnormalities or signs of inflammation. A fine-needle aspirate failed to yield a definitive diagnosis. The cat was reexamined 2 years later with a significant increase in the extent of iris involvement. Secondary abnormalities included corneal edema, retinal and optic nerve atrophy and secondary glaucoma. On histopathology, the tumor was diagnosed as a Schwann cell variant of a peripheral nerve sheath tumor, similar to iridal spindle cell tumors recently described in the dog.

(Image courtesy of Paige M. Evans, DVM; Evans PM, Lynch GI, Dubielzig RR: Anterior uveal spindle cell tumor in a cat. *Vet Ophthalmol* 13(6):387-390, 2010.)

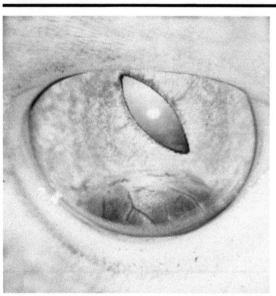

Figure 238
Neoplasia/Iridociliary leiomyoma
(adult domestic shorthair)

The owners were concerned about a change in iris color, noted a few days prior to examination. No pain or discharge had been noted. The ventrotemporal iris is relatively featureless and gray in color. Compare the surface texture of this area with that of the normal iris. Iris vessels are prominent at the lesion's dorsal margin and throughout the affected area. The iris base is displaced forward, compromising the anterior chamber and iridocorneal angle. Histopathologically, a ciliary body leiomyoma encroached upon the adjacent iris.

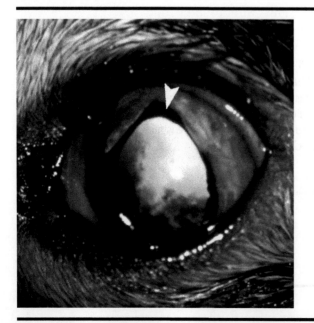

Figure 239
Neoplasia/Iridociliary leiomyosarcoma
(8-year-old domestic shorthair)

For 1 month, the owner had noticed a mild squint, with progressive depigmentation and swelling of the cat's iris. Normal iris structure is replaced peripherally by an elevated vascularized tissue. The pupillary iris is dark (*arrow*) and adheres to the lens. Axial anterior and posterior cortical cataracts are present. Direct pupillary light response (PLR) was negative, but the indirect PLR was positive. The fundus was normal. The cellular infiltrate in the iris and ciliary body was identified as a leiomyosarcoma.

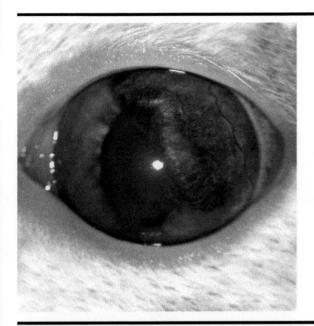

Figure 240
Neoplasia/Iridociliary leiomyosarcoma
(12-year-old domestic shorthair)

A change in iris color and the onset of squinting were noticed 1 week prior to presentation. From 11 o'clock to 4 o'clock, the iris appears dark gray and swollen, its surface extending well into the anterior chamber. Rubeosis causes the remaining iris to appear hyperemic. Its surface has a velvety appearance. Posterior synechia are accompanied by pigment hypertrophy along the pupillary margin. A moderate aqueous flare and diffuse fibrin formation alter anterior chamber clarity. The posterior segment could not be clearly visualized.

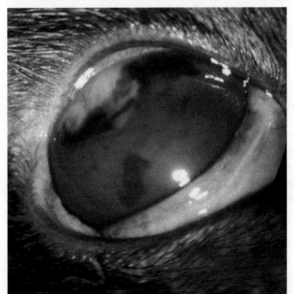

Figure 241
Neoplasia/Metastatic mammary adenocarcinoma
(16-year-old Siamese)

The cat began to squint its right eye a few days after surgical resection of multiple ulcerated mammary masses. Despite the presence of a mild anterior uveitis, the owner elected to observe the eye during the cat's post-operative convalescence. Over the course of 3 weeks, the eye became increasingly painful, as indicated by the prominent nictitans. A solid pale intraocular mass presses against the cornea at the temporal limbus. Intraocular detail is obscured by hemorrhage and fibrin. Metastatic mammary adenocarcinoma was confirmed histopathologically.

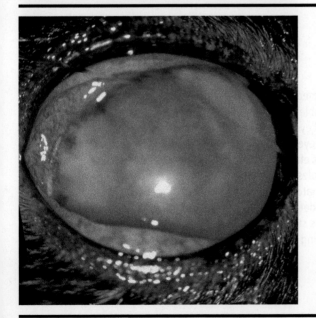

Figure 242
Neoplasia/Squamous cell carcinoma
(13-year-old domestic longhair)

Recently the eye had been becoming progressively cloudier and then acutely painful. The conjunctiva is hyperemic and chemotic. The severe corneal edema and perilimbal vascularization limit thorough evaluation of the anterior segment and fundus. Severe aqueous flare and fibrin also obscure intraocular detail. Intraocular pressure was moderately elevated. On ultrasound, the retina was totally detached. On histopathology, tumor cells were found in blood vessels throughout the entire uvea and into orbital tissue, leading to a diagnosis of metastatic squamous cell carcinoma. A primary site was not identified.

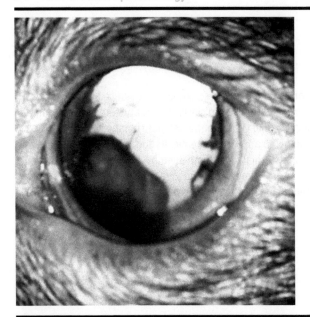

Figure 243
Neoplasia/Metastatic hemangiosarcoma
(1.5-year-old Siamese)

This cat was presented with a history of acute onset of lethargy and a red left eye. Ocular lesions were restricted to the anterior segment of the left eye and the posterior segment of the right (see Figure 377). A large, organized clot is present in the anterior chamber. Dark red tissue can be seen extending from the back of the iris through the dilated pupil. The cat died soon after examination and only the eyes were examined histopathologically. Lesions were due to metastatic hemangiosarcoma.

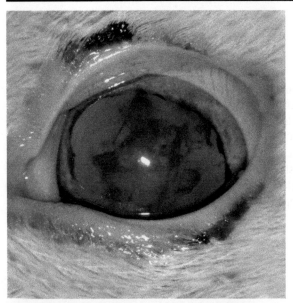

Figure 244
Neoplasia/Primitive neural epithelial tumor
(15-year-old domestic shorthair)

This cat was initially presented and treated for an anterior uveitis characterized by severe hyphema, miosis, and posterior synechia. The posterior segment was difficult to visualize at that time. The only positive laboratory result was a positive serologic test for *Bartonella henselae*. One month later, at the time of this photograph, the resting pupil is dilated and an irregularly shaped blood clot is centered in the pupillary space. It was now possible to detect a retinal detachment and associated atrophy. The globe was enucleated and submitted for histopathology. A mild lymphoplasmacytic inflammatory infiltrate was identified throughout the uvea. A neoplasm was found adjacent to the optic disc, extending the full thickness of the choroid and into the detached retina.

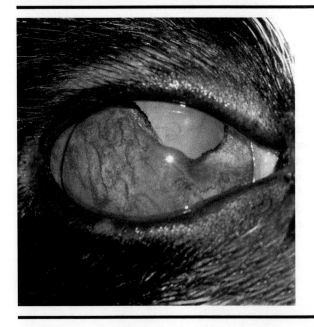

Figure 245
Neoplasia/Post-traumatic sarcoma
(8-year-old domestic shorthair)

This cat was adopted as a young adult. Ocular history prior to that time was unknown. No problems were seen until 4 weeks ago when the owner noted a prominent third eyelid and a localized change in iris color. By the time of examination, the eye had changed dramatically. A flesh-colored, highly vascularized mass effaces the temporal and ventral iris, distorting the pupil shape. Lens vacuoles are highlighted by the tapetal reflection, the latter dulled by inflammatory debris in the anterior vitreous and the presence of an exudative retinal detachment that spared only the mid-tapetal region of the fundus. No lesions suggestive of prior injury were identified. The diagnosis was made following enucleation and histopathologic examination.

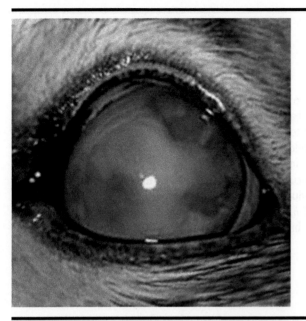

Figure 246
Neoplasia/Post-traumatic sarcoma
(12-year-old domestic shorthair)

Intermittent episodes of redness and squinting were reported following onset of a cataract at age 4. The owners seldom applied topical anti-inflammatory agents prescribed to treat lens-induced uveitis. Three years later, the owners relocated and presented the patient for examination. Findings on initial exam included corneal scarring, iritis, and a resorbing cataract. The patient was next seen 2 years later with a blind, painful eye attributed to active uveitis and a secluded pupil that prevented fundus examination. The owners declined enucleation. Eight months later, a fibrinohemorrhagic clot now obscures much of the inflamed iris. Perilimbal corneal scarring is present medially. Intraocular pressure is less than 5 mm Hg. Histopathologic examination of the enucleated globe confirmed the diagnosis. The cat was euthanized 7 months later when a sarcoma developed in the orbit.

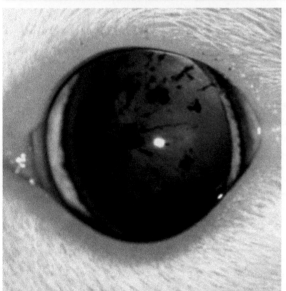

Figure 247
Post-inflammatory capsular cataract
(1-year-old domestic shorthair)

Several months prior to the photograph, this cat was treated for an anterior uveitis of undetermined etiology. Through the dilated pupil, large amounts of pigment can be seen deposited on the anterior lens capsule. There is also an anterior capsular and cortical cataract that further obscures the tapetal reflection.

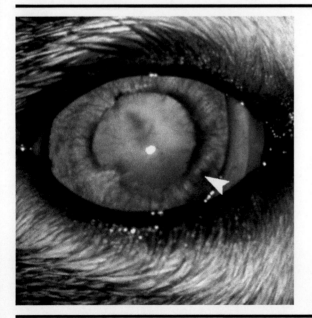

Figure 248
Posterior synechiae/Iris bombé/Secondary cataract
(16-year-old domestic shorthair)

For 10 months, this FeLV-positive cat had been treated for a bilateral anterior uveitis. The pupil is irregular because of circumferential posterior synechiae. Aqueous, now trapped in the posterior chamber, displaces the iris forward. The anterior chamber is shallow, especially nasally (*arrow*). Aqueous flare, an anterior capsular cataract and vitreous debris caused the mottled gray tapetal reflection.

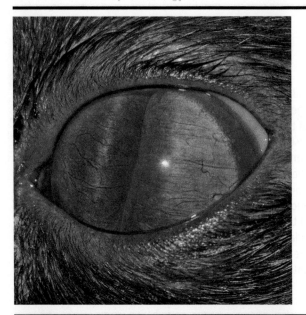

Figure 249
Iris bombé
(adult Siamese cross)

History was unknown in this adult stray. Two weeks ago, the foster owner noted an unusual appearing eye but saw no discharge or discomfort. Adhesions of iris to lens obstruct aqueous flow through the pupil, trapping fluid in the posterior chamber and displacing the iris forward. The iris face rests close to the inner corneal surface, effectively eliminating the anterior chamber. Iris vasculature is easily visualized in the thinned tissue. Perilimbal pigmentation is due to peripheral anterior synechiae and post-inflammatory pigment migration. Intraocular pressure (IOP) typically increases in patients with iris bombé, but IOP in this patient was within normal limits.

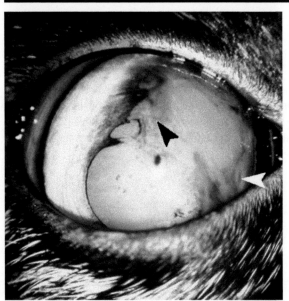

Figure 250
Posterior synechiae/Secondary cataract
(adult domestic shorthair)

After having been shot, several pellets were found in this cat's head and body, but none were identified within the globe or orbit. A dense corneal scar is present where a shot grazed the cornea (*white arrow*). As the inflammation resolved with treatment, a complete cataract formed. Posterior synechiae are present superiorly and nasally. Vascularization (*black arrow*) and pigment from the iris are present on the anterior lens surface.

SECTION VIII

Glaucoma

Atlas of Feline Ophthalmology. Second Edition. Kerry L. Ketring and Mary Belle Glaze.
© 2012 John Wiley & Sons, Inc. Published 2012 by John Wiley & Sons, Inc.

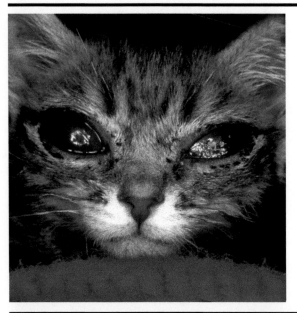

Figure 251
Congenital glaucoma
(4-week-old domestic shorthair)

This kitten was found on a farm by the owner. The kitten was totally blind but appeared otherwise healthy. Both globes are buphthalmic, with intraocular pressures of 60 mm Hg. The axial superficial ulcers are due to lagophthalmos and secondary exposure. Examination of the intraocular structures was difficult, but the pupil in the right eye appeared uniformly dilated with no signs of severe inflammation.

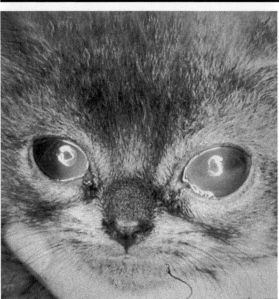

Figure 252
Congenital glaucoma
(4-week-old Persian)

This is one of three kittens in a litter, all buphthalmic at birth. The globes appear large, with generalized corneal opacification. Intraocular evaluation was limited by the corneal edema. The intraocular pressure was significantly elevated. Histopathology identified the expected sequelae of chronic glaucoma, as well as aniridia.

(Image courtesy of Milton Wyman, DVM, MS, DACVO.)

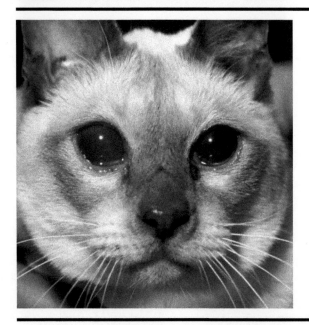

Figure 253
Inherited glaucoma
(12-year-old Siamese)

Presenting complaints included progressive vision loss and tearing over the past 3 months. Mild corneal edema is present superiorly. The pupils are dilated and nonresponsive. Both lenses are subluxated posteriorly and nasally. The optic discs appeared subjectively pale and depressed. The retinas were ophthalmoscopically normal. The intraocular pressure in the right eye was 44 mm Hg; in the left, 54 mm Hg. The cat is functionally blind.

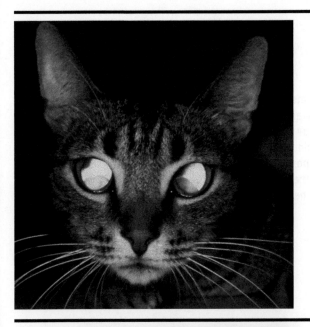

Figure 254
Inherited glaucoma
(4-year-old domestic shorthair)

The owners noted an increased tapetal reflection in both eyes. Both globes are mildly buphthalmic. Mild corneal edema is present bilaterally, especially in the ventral quadrant. The pupils are dilated and have a sluggish response to bright light. Both lenses are luxated posteriorly and inferiorly (see Figure 255). The optic discs were pale and surrounded by a zone of peripapillary retinal atrophy. The intraocular pressure in the right eye was 42 mm Hg; in the left, 26 mm Hg. No evidence of prior inflammation was present.

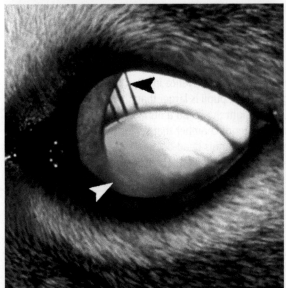

Figure 255
Inherited glaucoma
(4-year-old domestic shorthair)

This is a closer view of the left eye of the cat in Figure 254. Mild corneal edema is evident at the *white arrow*. Elongated ciliary processes (*black arrow*) extend toward the luxated lens. A large aphakic crescent is seen dorsally.

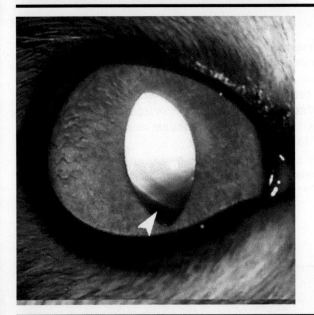

Figure 256
Primary open angle glaucoma (POAG)
(1-year-old domestic shorthair)

The owners noticed that the irises appeared odd and different from one another. A mild anisocoria was present. The remaining clinical signs were similar in both eyes. The anterior chamber is deeper than normal. A partial posterior lens luxation creates an aphakic crescent (*arrow*) in this right eye. Iridodonesis could be appreciated bilaterally. The IOP was 18 mm Hg OD and 19 mm Hg OS.

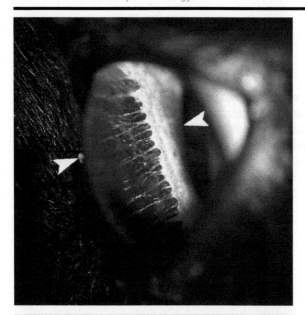

Figure 257
Primary open angle glaucoma (POAG)
(2-year-old domestic shorthair)

This cat was presented when its owners noted that one pupil was larger than the other. The lateral view of this left eye shows normal pectinate ligaments in an open drainage angle. The deep anterior chamber (between the *arrows*) is secondary to mild buphthalmia and a posterior lens luxation. Iridodonesis accompanied the posterior luxation in both eyes. IOP in the left eye was 32 mm Hg and in the right eye was 24 mm Hg. The right eye was functionally blind due to optic nerve atrophy, but the left eye was still visual at this time.

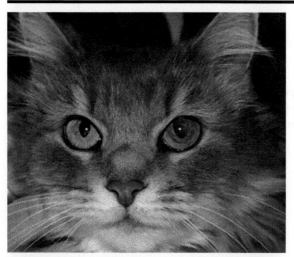

Figure 258
Feline aqueous humor misdirection syndrome (FAHMS)
(12-year-old domestic shorthair)

The owners had recently noticed a difference in pupil size and in the pupils' response to bright light. The left pupil is larger than the right, with a sluggish direct and indirect PLR. The right pupil had a normal direct and sluggish indirect PLR. The shallow anterior chamber that serves as a hallmark of FAHMS is not easily visualized in this head-on view of the left eye. There is also an anterior cortical cataract in the left lens. The IOP was 31 mm Hg OS and
18 mm Hg OD.

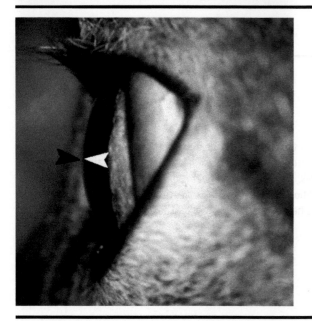

Figure 259
Feline aqueous humor misdirection syndrome (FAHMS)
(8-year-old Persian)

A veterinarian referred this animal for assessment of anisocoria. The left pupil was slightly larger than the right, but the pupillary reflexes remained within normal limits. The left iris and lens are displaced anteriorly. The anterior chamber between the cornea (*black arrow*) and the anteriorly displaced lens (*white arrow*) is extremely shallow (compare to Figure 5). The posterior segment is normal. Intraocular pressures measured 26 mm Hg in the right eye and 40 mm Hg in the left eye.

(Reproduced from *Veterinary Ocular Pathology: A Comparative Review*. Dubielzig, Ketring, McLellan, Albert. Elsevier Limited, 2010.)

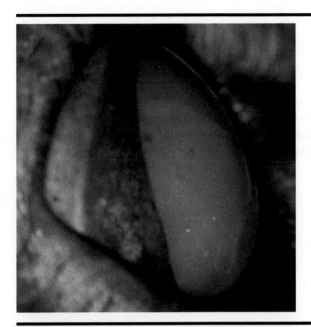

Figure 260
Feline aqueous humor misdirection syndrome (FAHMS)
(14-year-old domestic shorthair)

The owners were only aware of a progressive cataract in the right eye. The iris and lens are displaced anteriorly, as in Figure 259, although the shift is easier to appreciate with the densely opaque mature cataract. The IOP was difficult to accurately determine due to the proximity of the lens to the inner corneal surface. The right eye was similar in appearance to that of the cat in Figure 258.

(Reproduced from *Veterinary Ocular Pathology: A Comparative Review*. Dubielzig, Ketring, McLellan, Albert. Elsevier Limited, 2010.)

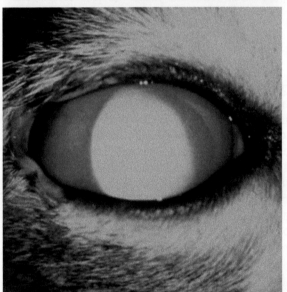

Figure 261
Congenital glaucoma
(10-week-old domestic shorthair)

The owners noticed a cloudy eye in this kitten. The right cornea is diffusely edematous and the pupil is nonresponsive to light. The posterior segment of both eyes showed no gross abnormalities. The intraocular pressure was 40 mm Hg in this eye and high normal in the opposite globe.

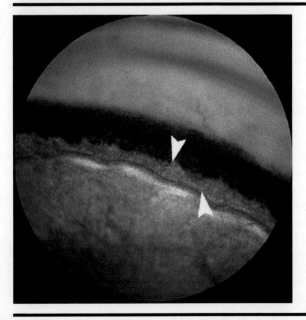

Figure 262
Anterior segment dysgenesis/Glaucoma
(10-week-old domestic shorthair)

The abnormal drainage angle in the left eye of the kitten in Figure 261 is seen through a Franklin goniolens. The pupil is located at the 6-o'clock position. The broad pigmented band represents sclera pigment. Normal pectinate ligaments are absent. Broad bands of iris tissue (*arrows*) span the angle. Compare this appearance to the normal angle in Figure 7.

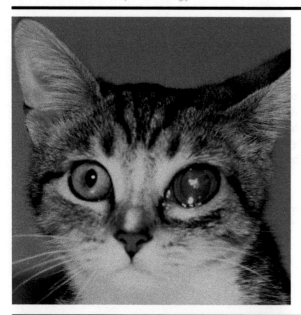

Figure 263
Secondary glaucoma
(6-month-old domestic shorthair)

Found as a stray, this kitten's right eye was normal. The left eye is buphthalmic with an IOP of 46 mm Hg. The pupil is dilated and nonresponsive and the iris is darkly pigmented. The optic nerve and retina were severely atrophic. On histopathology, a lymphoplasmacytic infiltrate was reported but no definitive etiology was found.

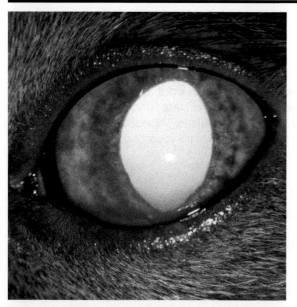

Figure 264
Secondary glaucoma/Post-inflammatory
(3-year-old Russian blue)

Presented due to cloudiness and squinting in the left eye, this cat's right eye was normal on examination. Corneal abnormalities include diffuse edema and keratic precipitates in the inferior quadrant. A moderate aqueous flare contributes to the general haziness. Rubeosis iridis and iris nodules replace the normal iris stroma. Fundus changes included optic disc pallor, generalized retinal atrophy, and perivascular cuffing. IOP at the time of this photograph was 38 mm Hg. The only significant laboratory result was a toxoplasmosis IgG titer of 1:1024. A generalized lymphoplasmacytic inflammatory infiltrate was found in the uvea, retina, and optic nerve head but no specific etiology was determined on histopathologic exam.

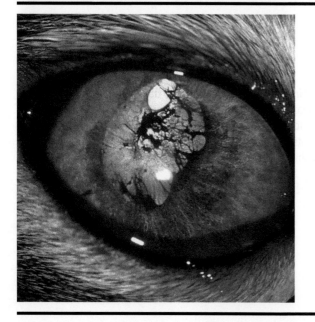

Figure 265
Secondary glaucoma/Post-inflammatory
(6-year-old domestic shorthair)

At 4 years of age, this cat was treated for a bilateral anterior uveitis of undetermined etiology. Excluding the cloudy pupil that resulted from the initial uveitis, no ocular problems had been noted since that time. During the past 6 months, his vision deteriorated and both eyes appeared to be increasing in size. There was no active inflammation at the time of this photograph. The pupils are dyscoric due to posterior synechia remaining from the prior inflammatory disease. The iris and lens in this eye are displaced anteriorly. The iridocorneal angle is further compromised by a broad peripheral anterior synechia. The IOP was 40 mm Hg in both eyes. The detail of the fundus was difficult to view, but atrophy of the optic nerve and retina were suspected.

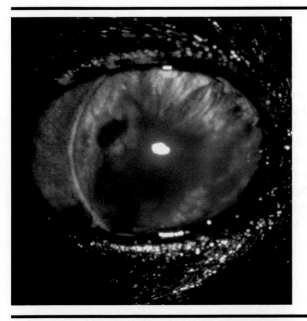

Figure 266
Secondary glaucoma/Hypertension
(20-year-old domestic shorthair)

Intraocular hemorrhage and blindness were the primary complaints in this patient. The right globe is mildly buphthalmic and the conjunctiva is hyperemic. A large blood clot is present, obscuring the miotic pupil. Circumferential adhesions of iris to lens trap aqueous within the posterior chamber. The resulting iris bombé results in a shallow anterior chamber that compromises iridocorneal angle form and function. The intraocular pressure was 36 mm Hg. The left eye also had hemorrhage in the anterior chamber and massive vitreous hemorrhage. The cat's mean systolic blood pressure was 280 mm Hg.

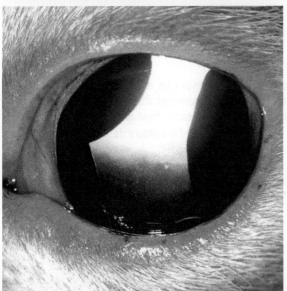

Figure 267
Secondary glaucoma/Iridociliary cysts
(12-year-old domestic shorthair)

Both eyes were similarly affected. The pupil in the left eye has been dilated with tropicamide to show the heavily pigmented iridociliary cysts. The cysts press the iris forward, decreasing the depth of the anterior chamber and reducing the ease of aqueous access into the iridocorneal angle. Over a 6-month period, the IOP increased to 28 mm Hg in both eyes.

(Reproduced from *Veterinary Ocular Pathology: A Comparative Review*. Dubielzig, Ketring, McLellan, Albert. Elsevier Limited, 2010.)

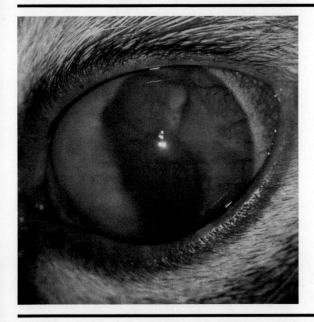

Figure 268
Secondary glaucoma/Lymphoma
(14-year-old domestic shorthair)

The owners were concerned that the left eye had changed from its normal blue color. Corneal edema and vascularization had progressed over a 3-month period. The iris is now orange in color, a consequence of stromal infiltrates and surface neovascularization. Blood-tinged fibrin obscures the pupil while diffuse posterior synechiae contribute to the dyscoria. The lens is diffusely opaque. Intraocular pressure was mildly elevated. Neoplastic cells were present throughout the uvea. Histopathologic changes in the optic nerve head and retina were compatible with glaucoma.

(Reproduced from *Veterinary Ocular Pathology: A Comparative Review*. Dubielzig, Ketring, McLellan, Albert. Elsevier Limited, 2010.)

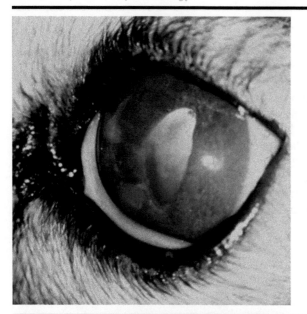

Figure 269
Secondary glaucoma/Feline diffuse iris melanoma
(12-year-old domestic shorthair)

This cat recently developed glaucoma but had undergone a change in iris color over the last several years. Diffuse iris thickening, increased pigmentation, and scattered surface nodules obscure normal iris detail. The pupillary margin adheres to the anterior lens surface. Both direct and indirect pupillary light reflexes are absent. Pigment can be seen on the anterior lens capsule. The optic disc was atrophic and retinal vessels were attenuated. The drainage angle could not be visualized because of anterior displacement of the iris. The intraocular pressure was greater than 60 mm Hg. Iris melanoma was confirmed histopathologically.

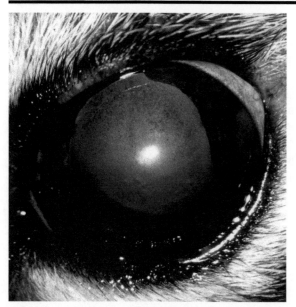

Figure 270
Secondary glaucoma/Feline diffuse iris melanoma
(12-year-old domestic shorthair)

This cat's iris had progressively darkened over a period of 8 years but only recently did the owners recognize a change in vision. Normal iris detail is obscured by the diffuse, dense pigmentation throughout the iris. The pupil is dilated, misshapen, and nonresponsive. Pigmentary debris is present across the anterior lens capsule. IOP was 60 mm Hg.

(Reproduced from *Veterinary Ocular Pathology: A Comparative Review*. Dubielzig, Ketring, McLellan, Albert. Elsevier Limited, 2010.)

SECTION IX

Lens

Atlas of Feline Ophthalmology. Second Edition. Kerry L. Ketring and Mary Belle Glaze.
© 2012 John Wiley & Sons, Inc. Published 2012 by John Wiley & Sons, Inc.

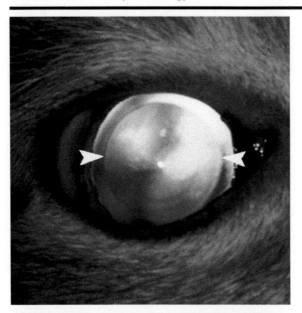

Figure 271
Senile nuclear sclerosis
(18-year-old domestic shorthair)

No visual deficit was noticed by the owners of this cat, presented for evaluation of cataracts. The pupil has been dilated to facilitate examination of the lens. The dense nucleus is clearly delineated (*arrows*) in the center of the lens. The tapetal reflection is easily seen and the fundus easily examined through the density.

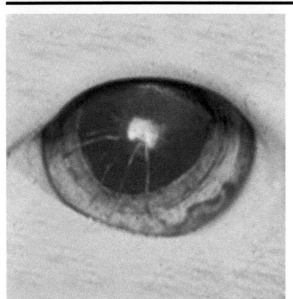

Figure 272
Capsular cataract/Persistent pupillary membranes (PPM)
(1-year-old domestic shorthair)

Multiple persistent pupillary membranes extend from the iris collarette to the anterior lens capsule where a distinct capsular opacity is seen. The PPMs were noted coincidentally when the cat was presented for evaluation of a corneal ulcer in the opposite eye. Progression of the capsular cataract is unlikely.

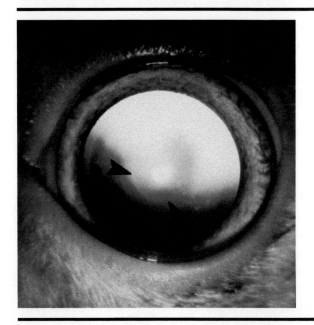

Figure 273
Nutritional cataract
(6-month-old Persian)

Born with a cleft palate, this kitten was raised on an unsupplemented milk substitute. The kitten has bilateral, posterior cortical, Y-suture opacities, which are difficult to visualize in the photograph. The perinuclear halo (*arrows*) is also compatible with an arginine-deficient diet.

(Image courtesy of J. Philip Pickett, DVM, DACVO.)

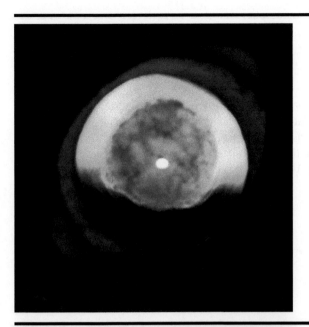

Figure 274
Nuclear cataract
(1.5-year-old domestic shorthair)

The pupil has been dilated for examination. The central cataract involves at least the embryonal and fetal nuclei at the core of the lens. The opacity obscures the tapetal reflection, appearing dark against the bright background. This examination technique, known as retroillumination, is an excellent method for detecting even subtle opacities in the normally clear ocular media. These bilateral cataracts did not progress during a 2-year follow-up.

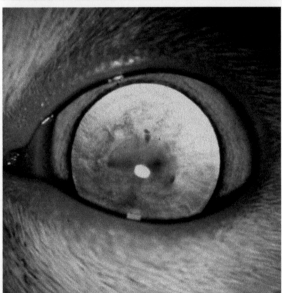

Figure 275
Immature cataract
(4-month-old Himalayan)

Bilateral cataracts were present in this kitten. Diffuse nuclear and cortical opacities are present, accounting for the decreased vision noted by the owners. The extent of the opacity is easily determined using the technique of retroillumination.

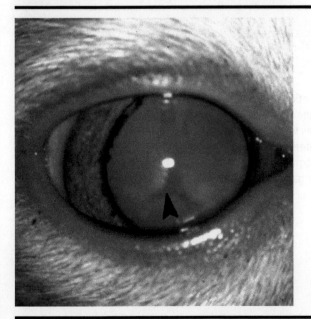

Figure 276
Hypermature cataract/Phacolytic uveitis
(5-month-old domestic shorthair)

This kitten is blind because of dense lens opacities in both eyes. The lens appears swollen and a widely separated suture line is evident (*arrow*). The iris is slightly hyperemic, and pigment from the posterior iris surface is seen on the lens capsule. Faint aqueous flare is also present.

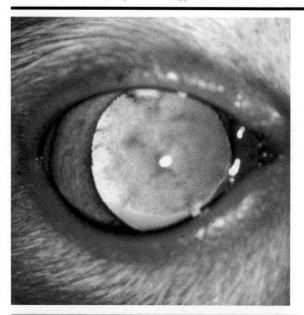

Figure 277
Resorbing cataract
(19-month-old domestic shorthair)

This is the same patient and the same eye as that depicted in Figure 276, only 14 months later. The lens diameter is decreasing as the cataract is resorbed, creating a deep anterior chamber and exposing the tapetal reflection around the lens circumference. Pigment deposits can be seen on the lens capsule. The cat is now able to see from both eyes.

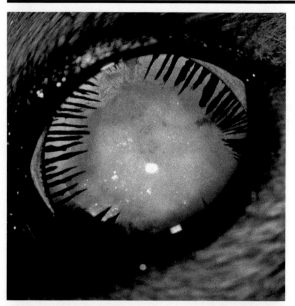

Figure 278
Resorbing cataract
(1-year-old domestic shorthair)

This stray cat had limited vision due to its bilateral ocular opacities. The pupil has been dilated for examination. The shrunken lens has a wrinkled capsule and a crystallized appearance that results from degraded lens fibers and protein within the resorbing cortical material. The ciliary processes encircle the lens and attach directly to the equatorial capsule. The eye shows little active inflammation. The normal retina could be visualized and the cat could follow objects when the pupils were dilated.

(Reproduced from *Veterinary Ocular Pathology: A Comparative Review*. Dubielzig, Ketring, McLellan, Albert. Elsevier Limited, 2010.)

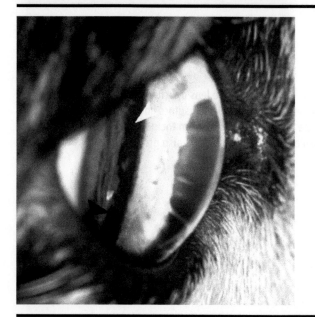

Figure 279
Resorbing cataract
(4-year-old domestic shorthair)

This cat was functionally visual despite a history of bilateral cataracts. This photograph of the right eye shows a deep anterior chamber, a consequence of decreased lens volume secondary to cataract resorption. The *black arrow* points to the anterior lens capsule, which is wrinkled. Although difficult to see in this photograph, the ciliary processes (*white arrow*) could be visualized in the gap created between the lens and iris.

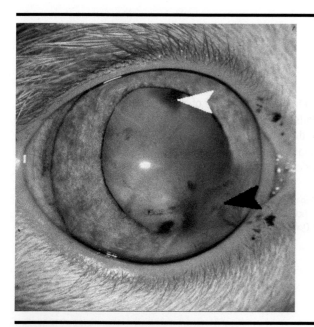

Figure 280
Anterior uveitis/Trauma
(2.5-year-old domestic shorthair)

The leukoma seen at the *black arrow* was thought to be the result of trauma sustained 6 months prior to the photograph. Corneal vascularization persists at the site. Mild aqueous flare accompanies a diffusely but subtly swollen iris. An anterior capsular and cortical cataract is present in the ventral half of the lens, aligned with the corneal lesion. The retina is totally detached and large blood clots can be seen in the vitreous (*white arrow*). Both the leukoma and cataract are presumably due to a penetrating injury. Routine serology failed to identify a cause beyond the presumed trauma. This eye is a prime candidate for post-traumatic sarcoma formation.

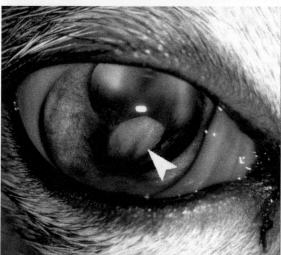

Figure 281
Post-traumatic lens resorption
(1.5-year-old domestic shorthair)

A leukoma at 6 o'clock and accompanying anterior and posterior synechiae were thought to be the result of a penetrating injury in this kitten. All that remains of the lens is a small dense remnant of cortical material (*arrow*). The retina was totally detached. Eleven years after this photograph, the eye was enucleated and diagnosed with a post-traumatic sarcoma.

(Reproduced from *Veterinary Ocular Pathology: A Comparative Review*. Dubielzig, Ketring, McLellan, Albert. Elsevier Limited, 2010.)

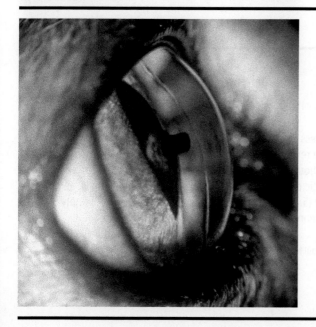

Figure 282
Lenticular foreign body
(adult domestic shorthair)

This cat presented with a complaint of chronic unilateral conjunctivitis. A more intriguing lesion was identified during examination of the opposite "normal" eye. A black, blunt cylindrical object protrudes into the anterior chamber from the central lens. A localized cataract and spots of capsular pigment surround the foreign body. A thin strand of mucus creates a vertical artifact across the corneal surface. No corneal scar could be identified as an entry point. The foreign body extended completely through the lens and also protruded into the anterior vitreous. Although no active inflammation is present in this visual eye, regular examinations were advised to watch for post-traumatic sarcoma formation, a potentially fatal neoplasm linked with lens damage in the cat.

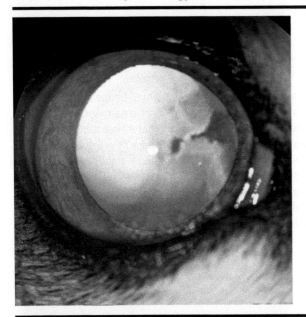

Figure 283
Immature cataract/*Encephalitozoon cuniculi*
(4-year-old European shorthair)

The owners presented this cat because of a color change in the right eye. A lens opacity extends from the anterior capsule and cortex to the nasal equatorial cortex, then continues into the posterior axial cortex. The cataract obscures the tapetal reflection in those areas. The fundus was normal. A small anterior cortical opacity was also identified in the left eye.

(Image courtesy of Barbara Nell DVM, DECVO; Benz P, MaaB G, Csokai J, Fuchs-Baumgartinger A, Schwendenwein I, Tichy A, Nell B: Detection of *Encephalitozoon cuniculi* in the feline cataractous lens. *Vet Ophthalmol* 14, Suppl 1:37-47, 2011.)

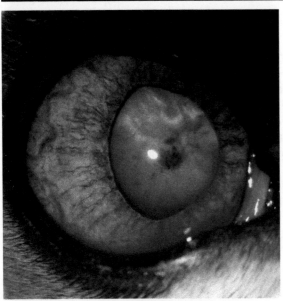

Figure 284
Hypermature cataract/*Encephalitozoon cuniculi*
(5-year-old European shorthair)

This is the same eye as in Figure 283, photographed 1 year later, and prior to phacoemulsification. Mild corneal edema is present inferiorly. The iris is diffusely swollen and ectropion uvea is present. Subtle aqueous flare accompanies pigmentary debris on the anterior lens capsule. A diffuse cataract obscures the tapetal reflection. *E. cuniculi* was identified histopathologically in the anterior cortex. PCR performed on the lens material was also positive for the parasite.

(Image courtesy of Barbara Nell DVM, DECVO; Benz P, MaaB G, Csokai J, Fuchs-Baumgartinger A, Schwendenwein I, Tichy A, Nell B: Detection of *Encephalitozoon cuniculi* in the feline cataractous lens. *Vet Ophthalmol* 14, Suppl 1:37-47, 2011.)

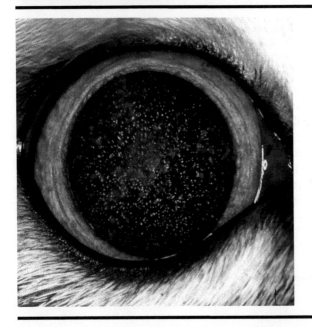

Figure 285
Hypocalcemic cataract
(2-year-old domestic shorthair)

Although weakness was this cat's primary symptom, initial physical examination also revealed bilateral cataracts. Fine punctate opacities are scattered throughout the anterior and posterior lens cortices. The cataracts were characteristic of those reported in hypocalcemic individuals; serum calcium was low (5.5 mg/dl). The metabolic changes were ultimately attributed to primary hypoparathyroidism.

(Image courtesy of Paul Miller, DVM, DACVO.)

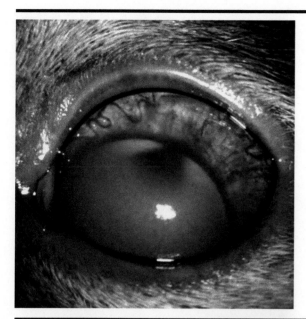

Figure 286
Anterior lens luxation
(9-year-old Siamese)

The owners complained of acute cloudiness and tearing in this patient's left eye. The entire lens is located within the anterior chamber. The localized corneal edema results from endothelial dysfunction following physical contact between the lens and inner corneal surface. Iris vessels are engorged and faint aqueous flare is present. The miotic pupil can be seen as a dark area just behind the upper lens. The intraocular pressure in this eye was subnormal; IOP in the right eye was within normal limits. This cat also had a subluxated lens in the right eye.

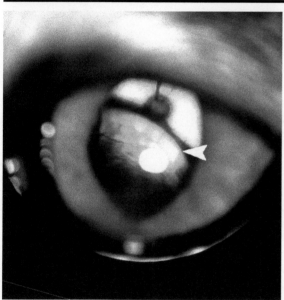

Figure 287
Posterior lens luxation
(4-year-old domestic shorthair)

This photograph is of the same eye depicted in Figures 254 and 255. The camera is focused on the pale optic disc and the surrounding retinal atrophy. The superior equator of the posteriorly luxated lens can be seen just out of the plane of focus (*arrow*).

SECTION X

Vitreous

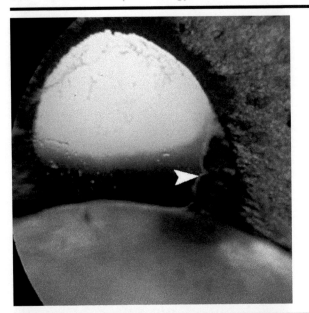

Figure 288
Anterior lens luxation/Persistent hyaloid
(2-year-old domestic shorthair)

This cat was presented for evaluation of a cloudy left eye. This close-up photograph shows the lens luxated into the anterior chamber. Only a small portion of the cloudy lens can be visualized occupying the lower half of the photo. A persistent hyaloid artery (*arrow*) is attached to the posterior lens surface. Intraocular pressure (IOP) was 20 mm Hg. The right eye was glaucomatous, with an IOP of 34 mm Hg and a posterior lens subluxation. Optic disc cupping was present in the right eye (see Figure 388).

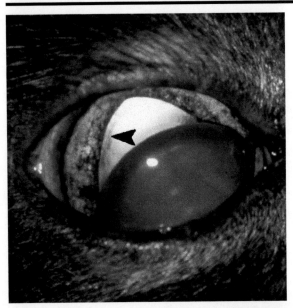

Figure 289
Hyalitis/Anterior lens luxation
(14-year-old domestic shorthair)

The owners were unaware of any prior ocular or systemic disease. The lens is luxated into the anterior chamber, resulting in mild corneal edema. Although pigmented, the iris appears normal. A mild hyalitis is present (*arrow*). The left eye also had an anteriorly luxated lens and hyalitis. The intraocular pressure was 48 mm Hg in the right eye and 20 mm Hg in the left. The cat was positive for FIV but negative for FeLV and *Toxoplasma gondii*.

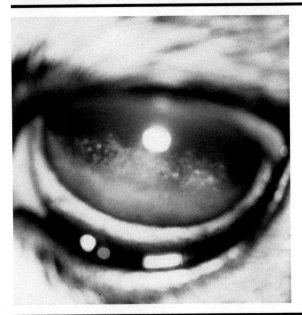

Figure 290
Hyalitis/Pars planitis/Toxoplasmosis
(6-year-old domestic shorthair)

The owners were concerned about the development of a darker left iris in their cat. All ocular lesions were restricted to the left eye and included mild aqueous flare, keratic precipitates, and iris congestion. The pupil has been dilated in this photograph. Inflammatory cells suspended in the anterior vitreous appear as a white flocculent material posterior to the iris, following the curvature of the posterior lens. Serology for FIV and FeLV was negative. The toxoplasmosis titer was positive at 1:512 IgM and 1:12,048 IgG.

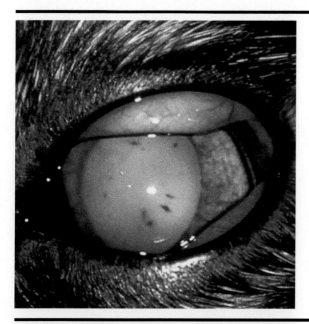

Figure 291
Hyalitis
(7-year-old domestic shorthair)

This cat had been treated for anterior uveitis for 3 weeks. The conjunctiva is chemotic. Faint aqueous flare is present, as are pigment deposits on the anterior lens capsule. The dull yellow color seen through the pupil is the result of abundant cellular infiltrates within the vitreous. All serology was negative. Pyogranulomatous panophthalmitis of unknown etiology was identified on histopathologic exam.

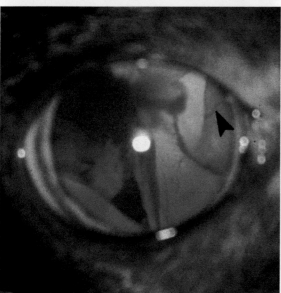

Figure 292
Vitreous hemorrhage/Hypertension
(14-year-old Siamese)

Presented for acute blindness of 1 week's duration, this cat had bilateral bullous retinal detachments and vitreous hemorrhage. The hemorrhage is easily seen through the dilated pupil. A retinal vessel (*arrow*) can be seen as a consequence of the detached retina. The systolic blood pressure was 240 mm Hg.

SECTION XI

Retina and Choroid

Atlas of Feline Ophthalmology. Second Edition. Kerry L. Ketring and Mary Belle Glaze.
© 2012 John Wiley & Sons, Inc. Published 2012 by John Wiley & Sons, Inc.

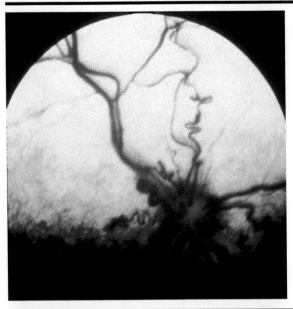

Figure 293
Cardiovascular anomalies
(6-month-old domestic shorthair)

Cyanosis and exercise intolerance were chronic problems for this kitten. On cardiac auscultation, individual heart sounds could not be distinguished because of a continual "machinery" murmur. The retinal vessels are distended and tortuous. Both eyes were similarly affected. Cardiomegaly and multiple septal defects were identified at necropsy.

(Image courtesy of Lorraine G. Karpinski, VMD, DACVO.)

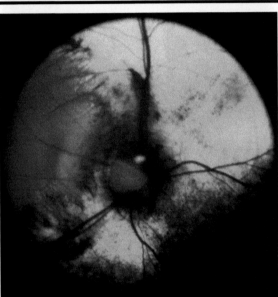

Figure 294
Scleral coloboma
(6-month-old domestic shorthair)

This is the fundus of the eye pictured in Figure 33. A large sclera coloboma appears as a pale area to the left of the optic disc. The defect extends into the area of the lamina cribrosa, also altering the optic nerve head.

(Reproduced from *Veterinary Ocular Pathology: A Comparative Review*. Dubielzig, Ketring, McLellan, Albert. Elsevier Limited, 2010.)

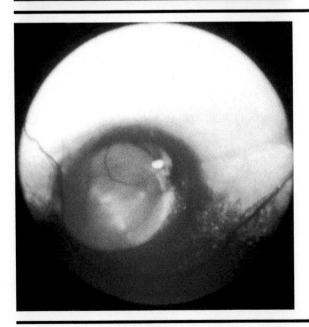

Figure 295
Scleral coloboma
(14-year-old domestic shorthair)

This was a coincidental finding on routine examination. The photograph of the temporal fundus is taken through a 28-diopter lens. The rim of the optic disc is just visible at the 3-o'clock position. The white circular lesion represents a posteriorly recessed scleral pocket. Retinal vessels course over the rim of the depression and across the defect. Although the lesion is surrounded by a border of dark choroidal pigment, the choroid within the defect is hypoplastic.

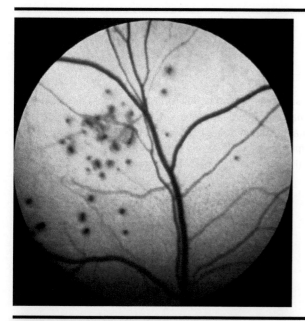

Figure 296
Retinal dysplasia
(5-month-old Abyssinian)

Presented for the evaluation of an extensive symblepharon in one eye, this kitten also had bilateral congenital retinal lesions. The dark foci are the result of folds in the outer retinal layers. In this patient, the lesions have a subtly reflective border and are restricted to the tapetal region.

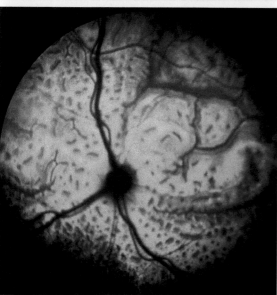

Figure 297
Retinal dysplasia
(4-month-old domestic shorthair)

This cat had bilateral congenital cataracts. The photograph is of the fundus of the now aphakic left eye following lens extraction. Congenital retinal folds appear as dark spots and branching lines that obscure the underlying tapetum. Dysplasia is a common finding in cats with congenital cataracts.

(Reproduced from *Veterinary Ocular Pathology: A Comparative Review*. Dubielzig, Ketring, McLellan, Albert. Elsevier Limited, 2010.)

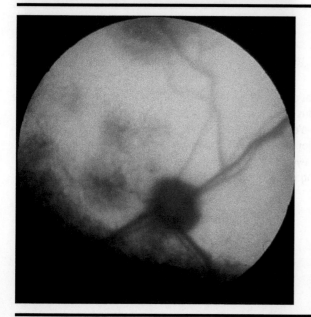

Figure 298
Chorioretinitis/Feline leukemia complex
(10.5-year-old domestic shorthair)

This is the right fundus of the cat with anterior uveitis pictured in Figure 180. Focal areas of abnormal pigment proliferation and edema are present in the tapetal retina. This cat was FeLV positive.

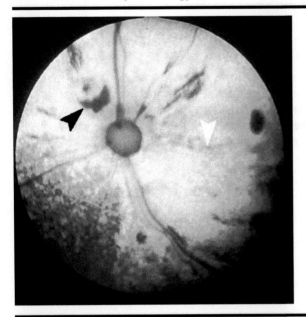

Figure 299
Chorioretinitis/Feline leukemia complex
(4-year-old domestic shorthair)

Bilateral retinal lesions were found in this cat presented with a complaint of lethargy. The retinal vessels appear pale and thready as a consequence of anemia. Deep intraretinal hemorrhage (*black arrow*) and superficial flame-shaped hemorrhage (*white arrow*) within the nerve fiber layer can be seen throughout the fundus. Feline leukemia virus infection was diagnosed by serology.

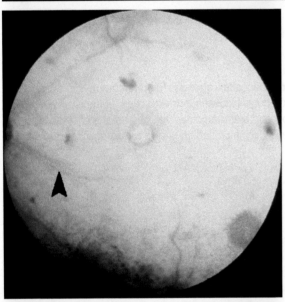

Figure 300
Chorioretinitis/Feline leukemia complex
(2.5-year-old domestic shorthair)

This cat was presented for examination because of listlessness and anorexia. The left temporal tapetal retina has focal retinal hemorrhages, Other areas of abnormal tapetal coloration represent edema or prior hemorrhage. The retinal vessels (*arrow*) are extremely attenuated because of the severe anemia (packed cell volume = 7%). The very edge of the optic disc can be seen at 9 o'clock. Feline leukemia virus infection was diagnosed by serology.

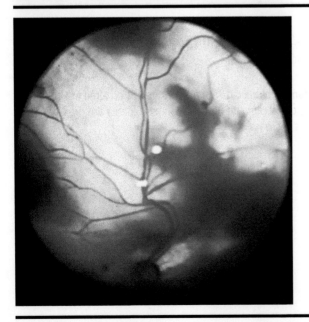

Figure 301
Chorioretinitis/Feline leukemia complex
(6-year-old domestic shorthair)

The sudden onset of poor vision led to this patient's examination. This image of the right fundus was taken through a 28-diopter lens. The optic disc is located at the 6-o'clock position. Massive subretinal hemorrhage elevates the retina superior to the optic disc, altering the course of the overlying vessels. The left eye had a total retinal detachment. The only significant laboratory finding was a positive test for feline leukemia virus.

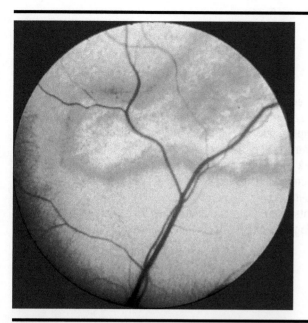

Figure 302
Chorioretinopathy/Panleukopenia
(2-year-old domestic shorthair)

This adult cat was presented with ataxia due to cerebellar hypoplasia. The well-circumscribed area of altered tapetal reflectivity is reminiscent of the retinal disorganization and degeneration seen as a consequence of experimentally induced feline panleukopenia.

(Image courtesy of Alan D. MacMillan, DVM, PhD, DACVO.)

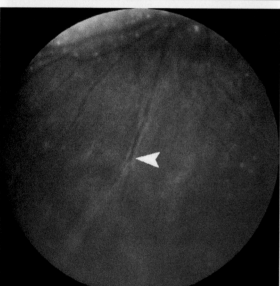

Figure 303
Chorioretinitis/Feline infectious peritonitis
(7-year-old domestic shorthair)

This is the left posterior segment of the cat featured in Figure 193. Perivascular cuffing (*arrow*) and focal intraretinal exudates are present. The only positive laboratory results were a high titer for feline coronavirus and an elevated total blood protein.

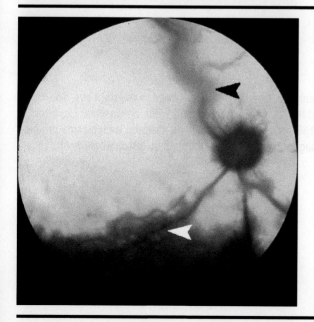

Figure 304
Chorioretinitis/Feline infectious peritonitis
(3-year-old domestic shorthair)

A painful left eye and a history of lethargy led to this cat's presentation. The left eye had a severe anterior uveitis and its posterior segment could not be visualized. In the right fundus, perivascular exudates (*arrows*) blur the detail of dilated retinal vessels within the nerve fiber layer. Postmortem histopathology confirmed the diagnosis.

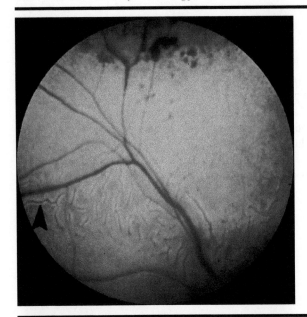

Figure 305
Retinal folds/Feline infectious peritonitis
(10-month-old Himalayan)

The owners reported seizures of increasing frequency and severity over a 6-hour period. The anterior segment was unremarkable with the exception of sluggish, incomplete pupillary light reflexes. The edge of the optic disc can be seen at the ventral limit of the photograph. Multiple retinal folds (*arrow*) appear as thin dark lines throughout the tapetal fundus. The margin of a large subretinal hemorrhage is seen dorsally, flanked by smaller preretinal and intraretinal hemorrhages. The cat's vision was difficult to assess owing to his altered mentation. He was euthanized as his neurologic status deteriorated. A diagnosis of FIP was confirmed at necropsy.

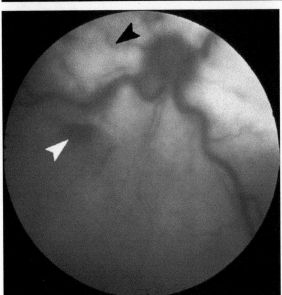

Figure 306
Chorioretinitis/Feline infectious peritonitis
(1.5-year-old Siamese)

For 1 week, this cat had been listless, febrile, and anorectic. Bilateral anterior uveitis was characterized by moderate aqueous flare and large cellular precipitates within the anterior chamber. Retinal vessels are notably dilated on funduscopic examination. Subretinal edema elevates the retina, blurring underlying structural detail. Subretinal hemorrhage (*white arrow*) and perivascular exudates (*black arrow*) can be seen. The majority of the red color is due to reflection from normal choroidal vessels easily seen in this color-dilute breed. FIP was suspected based on a total plasma protein of 9.9 g/dl with a 4.37 g/dl gamma globulin.

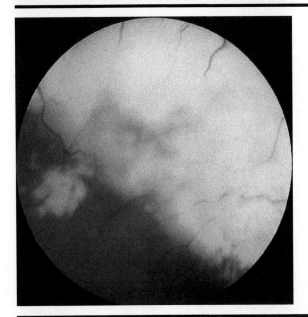

Figure 307
Chorioretinitis/Feline infectious peritonitis
(8-month-old domestic shorthair)

The cat was presented with severe anterior uveitis in the right eye. The temporal retina of the left eye is elevated and white perivascular exudates are present. A 1:1600 coronavirus titer and an elevated total plasma protein level led to the diagnosis, which was confirmed by histopathology at necropsy.

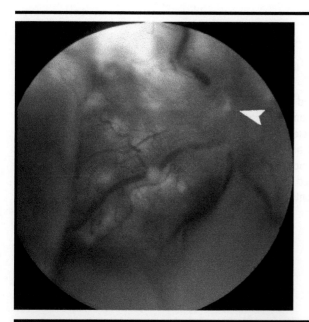

Figure 308
Chorioretinitis/Feline infectious peritonitis
(5-year-old domestic shorthair)

This is the left eye of the cat in Figure 196. This retina is totally detached and the retinal vessels are dilated. Perivascular and subretinal exudates are present in the center of the photograph. The optic disc (*arrow*) is obscured by exudates.

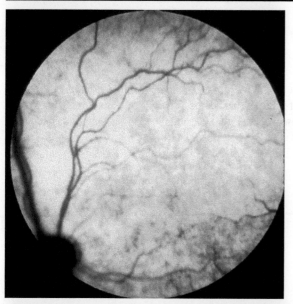

Figure 309
Chorioretinitis/Histoplasmosis
(5-year-old domestic shorthair)

This cat had respiratory problems for 2 weeks and was increasingly dyspneic. Body temperature was 100.5°F. The spleen and liver were enlarged. This photograph, taken with a neutral density filter, shows a mottled, pigmented tapetum. *Histoplasma capsulatum* organisms were found in the lung, liver, spleen, and outer layers of the retina, choroid, and sclera.

(Image courtesy of Art J. Quinn, DVM, DACVO.)

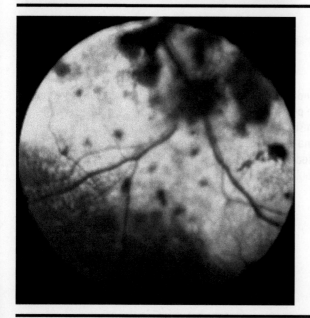

Figure 310
Chorioretinitis/Histoplasmosis
(2-year-old domestic shorthair)

This young adult cat presented with a 3-week history of lethargy and weight loss. Harsh inspiratory lung sounds and fever were noted on physical examination. Multifocal darkly colored exudates obscure the tapetal reflection near the optic nerve. Smaller pigmented foci and retinal hemorrhages are scattered throughout. The optic disc is dark and poorly defined in this blind eye. The diagnosis was confirmed when *H. capsulatum* was identified in a lymph node aspirate.

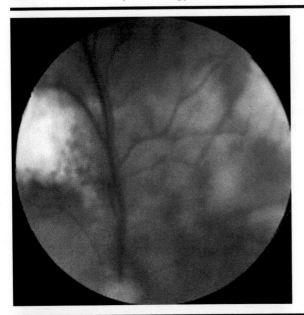

Figure 311
Chorioretinitis/Histoplasmosis
(7-year-old Domestic shorthair)

This cat's pupils had been dilated for several weeks before the owner noted a change in its vision. Occasional sneezing was also reported. Extensive subretinal gray to cream-colored exudates obscure the tapetal reflection. The retina is detached, accounting for the vision loss. Anterior segment inflammation was not present at this initial examination, but severe anterior uveitis accompanied a relapse of ocular signs when antifungal therapy was discontinued 6 months later. Vision never improved.

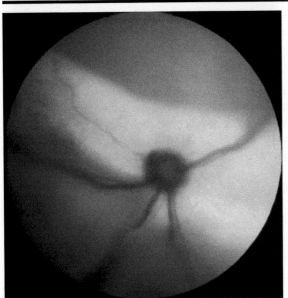

Figure 312
Chorioretinitis/Histoplasmosis
(8-year-old domestic shorthair)

This is the fundus of the cat in Figures 68 and 204. The entire inferior retina is elevated because of subretinal exudates. A large detachment is also present superiorly. *Histoplasma capsulatum* was identified in the subretinal exudate.

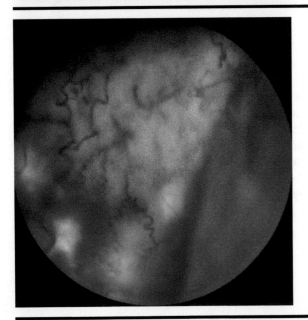

Figure 313
Chorioretinitis/Histoplasmosis
(1.5-year-old domestic shorthair)

This is the right fundus of the cat pictured in Figure 90. The anterior segment in this eye and the posterior segment of the left eye were normal. A large intraretinal and presumed subretinal granuloma is present superiorly, and the remaining retina is detached. The optic disc cannot be visualized. The diagnosis was based on the presence of *Histoplasma* organisms within the biopsy of the left bulbar conjunctival mass.

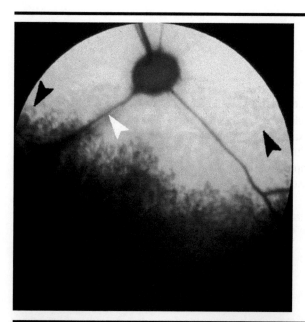

Figure 314
Chorioretinitis/Cryptococcosis
(11-year-old domestic shorthair)

This is the fundus of the cat in Figure 207. The tapetum has a mottled appearance due to focal edema (*black arrows*). There is one area of perivascular exudate at the white arrow.

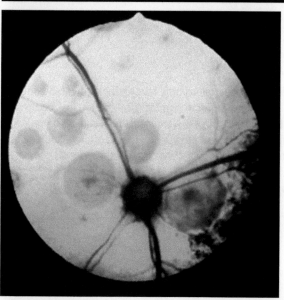

Figure 315
Chorioretinitis/Cryptococcosis
(6-year-old domestic shorthair)

Lethargy, poor appetite, and chronic nasal discharge were presenting complaints in this patient. The anterior segments of both eyes were normal. Chorioretinitis is characterized by multifocal circles of well-defined subretinal edema that surround darker granulomatous central exudates. An aspirate from a small mass in the left nostril revealed cryptococcal organisms on cytology.

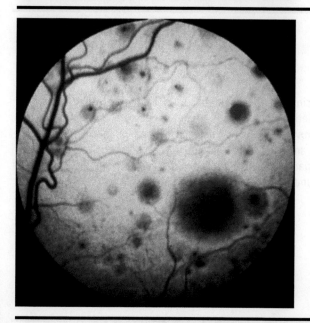

Figure 316
Chorioretinitis/Cryptococcosis
(5-year-old domestic shorthair)

Broad-spectrum antibiotics had no effect on this cat's nasal discharge of 3 months' duration. The anterior segments of both eyes were normal. The retinal vessels are distended, with notable arteriolar tortuosity. Retinal and subretinal exudates appear as multiple pigmented foci throughout the tapetal fundus. *Cryptococcus neoformans* was detected in a bone marrow aspirate, confirming a positive serologic titer.

(Image courtesy of Art J. Quinn, DVM, DACVO.)

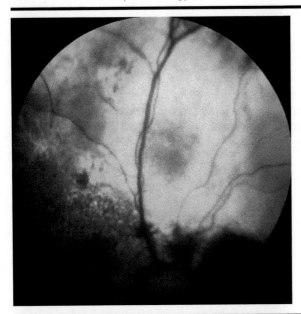

Figure 317
Chorioretinitis/Cryptococcosis
(5-year-old domestic shorthair)

This is the fundus of the cat in Figure 208. Both eyes were similarly affected. The multiple ill-defined grey areas represent subretinal and choroidal granulomatous exudates. Elevation of retinal vessels can be appreciated at the 3-o'clock position. The optic disc appears dark due to photographic technique. Dark areas of abnormal pigmentation can be seen immediately superior to the disc.

(Reproduced from *Veterinary Ocular Pathology: A Comparative Review*. Dubielzig, Ketring, McLellan, Albert. Elsevier Limited, 2010.)

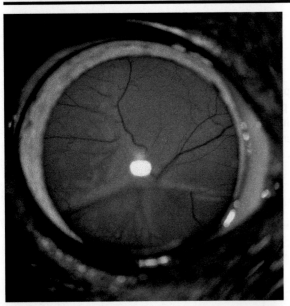

Figure 318
Retinal Detachment/Cryptococcosis
(11-year-old domestic shorthair)

This cat developed multiple cutaneous nodules after being treated with oral prednisolone for 1 month to control its asthma. Acute vision loss occurred shortly thereafter. Both eyes in this cat were similarly affected. The retina is totally detached and retinal vessels are apparent just posterior to the lens. Focal and linear exudates appear pale beneath the retinal vessels. No tapetal reflex can be seen because of the severe choroiditis. The diagnosis was confirmed on histopathology of the skin and ocular lesions.

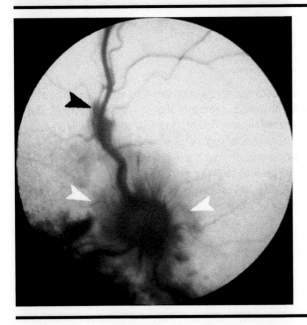

Figure 319
Chorioretinitis/Cryptococcosis
(4-year-old domestic shorthair)

Both eyes were similarly affected in this cat, presented because of lethargy and blindness. Retinal hemorrhages are present below the superior retinal venule (*black arrow*) and in the peripapillary nerve fiber layer. The optic nerve is swollen and the peripapillary retina is elevated (*white arrows*). *Cryptococcus* organisms were identified in the choroid, subretinal space, and meninges surrounding the optic nerve.

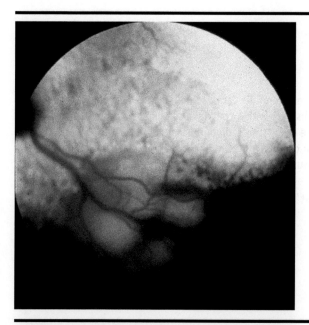

Figure 320
Chorioretinitis/Blastomycosis
(3-year-old domestic shorthair)

Dyspnea, depression, and elevated body temperature accompanied ocular lesions in this cat, which was lost for 5 days and found disoriented 2 days prior to admission. The retina at the tapetal-nontapetal junction is elevated by a cream-colored, granulomatous exudate, suggestive of mycotic chorioretinitis. Scattered pigment and altered reflectivity characterize the tapetum superior to the granuloma. The cat died approximately 24 hours after hospitalization. Large numbers of *Blastomyces dermatitidis* organisms were found within the ciliary body, choroid, and tapetum.

(Image courtesy of Mark Nasisse, DVM, DACVO; Nasisse M: Ocular changes in a cat with systemic blastomycosis. *JAVMA* 187:629, 1985.)

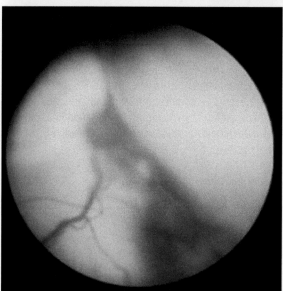

Figure 321
Chorioretinitis/Blastomycosis
(4-year-old domestic shorthair)

This outdoor cat was presented for evaluation when the owner noted its poor appetite and accompanying weight loss. Non-ocular abnormalities included fever, mild dyspnea, and a draining skin lesion on the right hind paw. The anterior segments of both eyes were normal. Posteriorly, the optic disc and one main retinal vessel are recognizable but a complete exudative retinal detachment obscures the remaining fundus detail. A cream-colored subretinal exudate is visible at 5 o'clock. This eye is blind. The opposite eye was less severely affected and remained sighted. The organism was identified cytologically in a sample from the skin lesion.

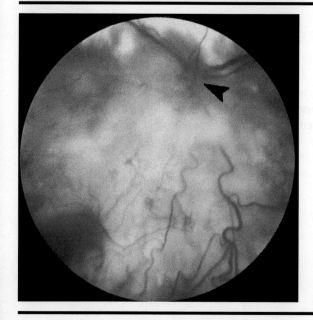

Figure 322
Chorioretinitis/Blastomycosis
(11-year-old domestic longhair)

Blindness was this cat's presenting complaint. A massive granulomatous exudate appears pinkish white, obscuring fundus detail. The majority of the cellular material is subretinal, separating the retina from the underlying choroid. Preretinal exudates obscure retinal vessels near the optic disc (*arrow*). Scattered hemorrhages and dilated, tortuous blood vessels are also seen above the exudates. The suspicion of mycotic disease was confirmed at necropsy.

(Image courtesy of Art J. Quinn, DVM, DACVO.)

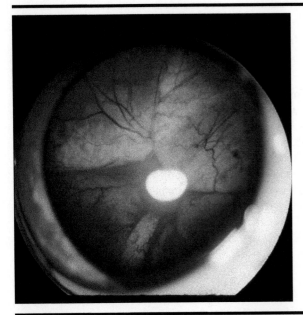

Figure 323
Chorioretinitis/Coccidioidomycosis
(2-year-old domestic shorthair)

A sibling and housemate of the cat pictured in Figure 211, this cat was presented 2 months later with a complaint of blindness. There were no signs of systemic disease or anterior segment ocular involvement. This photograph, taken through a dilated pupil, shows a complete retinal detachment with subretinal exudates and focal retinal hemorrhage.

(Image courtesy of Paul M. Barrett, DVM, DACVO.)

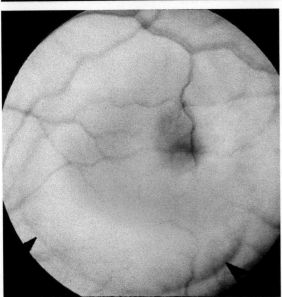

Figure 324
Chorioretinitis/Coccidioidomycosis
(2-year-old domestic shorthair)

This is the opposite fundus of the cat in Figure 323. The darker central area in the peripheral retina represents an early subretinal granuloma. Adjacent changes in tapetal coloration and reflectivity represent retinal edema and the edge of an early bullous detachment (*arrows*). An immunodiffusion test for *Coccidioides immitis* was positive.

(Image courtesy of Paul M. Barrett, DVM, DACVO.)

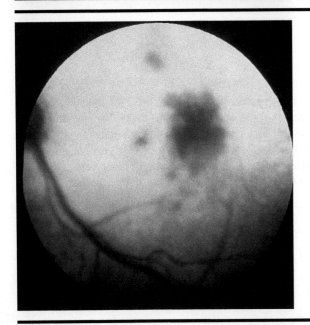

Figure 325
Chorioretinitis/Toxoplasmosis
(5.5-year-old domestic shorthair)

This cat was diagnosed with toxoplasmosis based on an IgG titer of 1:4096. The optic disc is just visible at the photograph's left margin. Near the area centralis is a subretinal exudate with satellite foci of edema and abnormal pigment.

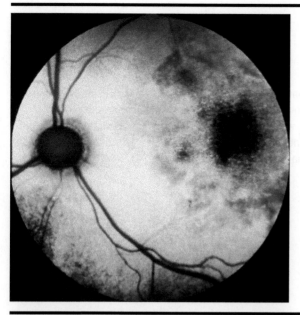

Figure 326
Chorioretinopathy/Toxoplasmosis
(6-year-old domestic shorthair)

This is the same cat in Figure 325, examined 5 months later. Active inflammation has resolved. Pigmentation of the tapetal fundus is a conspicuous sequela. Post-inflammatory retinal atrophy contributes to the surrounding tapetal hyperreflectivity.

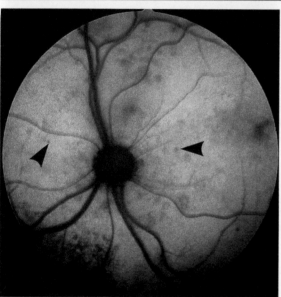

Figure 327
Chorioretinitis/Toxoplasmosis
(12-year-old domestic shorthair)

Presented for unilateral anterior uveitis, this cat also had bilateral retinal lesions. Pinpoint intraretinal hemorrhages are present (*arrows*). Intraretinal and subretinal exudates appear as dark foci adjacent to the optic disc and scattered throughout the tapetal retina. Toxoplasmosis titers were positive: IgM was 1:64 and IgG was 1:256.

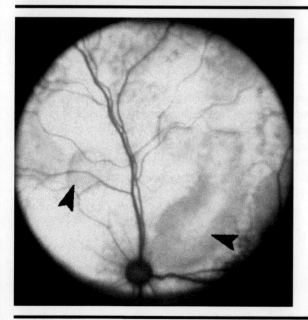

Figure 328
Chorioretinitis/Toxoplasmosis
(6-year-old Manx)

Toxoplasmosis had been diagnosed as the cause of a unilateral anterior uveitis 18 months beforehand. Multiple bullous retinal detachments now alter tapetal reflectivity (*arrows*). Fundus structures appear small in this photograph, taken through a 28-diopter lens. The only positive serology was a toxoplasmosis IgM titer of 1:64 and an IgG titer of 1:2048.

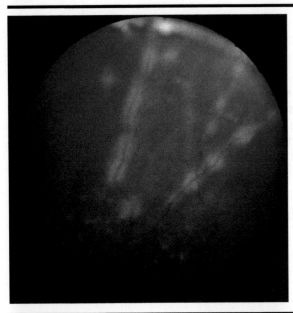

Figure 329
Chorioretinitis/Toxoplasmosis
(9-year-old domestic shorthair)

Presented for evaluation of a cloudy left eye, this cat was diagnosed with an exudative anterior uveitis. The ipsilateral nontapetal retina shows perivascular cuffing and focal intraretinal and preretinal exudates. Tests for FeLV and FIP were negative. A toxoplasmosis titer was positive at 1:256. The right eye was normal.

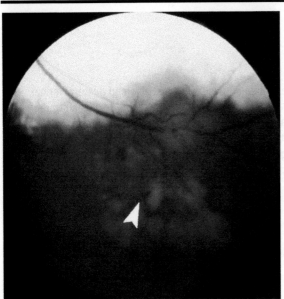

Figure 330
Chorioretinitis/Toxoplasmosis
(5.5-year-old domestic shorthair)

The right eye had a severe anterior uveitis that prevented examination of the retina. In the left eye, a granulomatous exudate obscures retinal vessels in the nontapetal region. Focal intraretinal hemorrhage (*arrow*) is also present. The only positive laboratory finding was a low *Toxoplasma* titer that was not repeated.

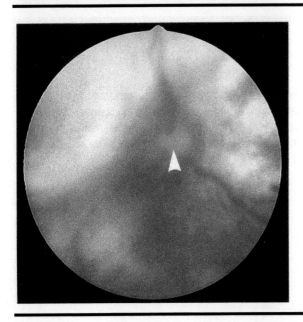

Figure 331
Chorioretinitis/Toxoplasmosis
(9-year-old domestic shorthair)

This cat went acutely blind after a 1-month period of lethargy, anorexia and weight loss. The pupils were dilated and unresponsive. The anterior segments had only a mild aqueous flare. A subretinal exudate elevates the left retina and obscures underlying tapetal detail. Pigment proliferates around the swollen optic disc (*arrow*). Similar changes were present in the right fundus. An FIV test was positive, as were titers for toxoplasmosis (IgM of 1:128; IgG of 1:2048).

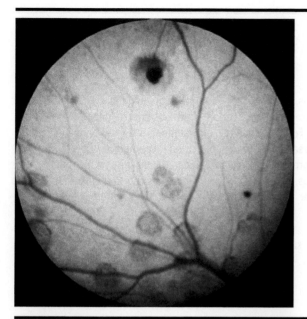

Figure 332
Chorioretinitis/*Feline hemotropic mycoplasmosis*
(1-year-old domestic shorthair)

This cat was icteric and in respiratory distress when presented for examination. Intraretinal hemorrhages appear as small red dots throughout the tapetal fundus. The dark circular lesions are presumably sites of previous hemorrhage. The cat had a regenerative anemia and was FeLV negative. *Mycoplasma haemofelis* (previously termed *Haemobartonella felis)* was diagnosed on a direct blood smear.

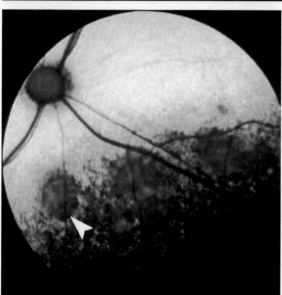

Figure 333
Retinitis/Bacterial meningitis
(6.5-year-old domestic shorthair)

This cat was presented with a history of acute blindness 48 hours prior to examination. Both pupils were dilated and nonresponsive. The only lesions were rounded areas of altered coloration along the tapetal junction. These areas of retinitis had pink centers, presumably due to cellular infiltrates, with grey and pigmented borders. All routine serology was negative. A cerebral spinal fluid tap yielded a culture of *Enterococcus avium*. Vision returned following antibiotic therapy.

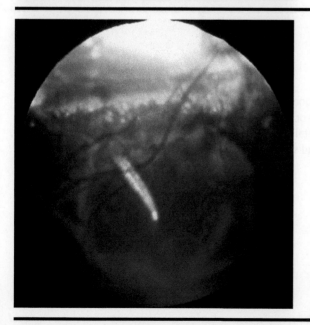

Figure 334
Chorioretinitis/Ophthalmomyiasis
(18-month-old domestic shorthair)

Presented because of inspiratory dyspnea, this cat had a lack of menace response and incomplete pupillary light reflexes. The white segmented body of a fly larva is located beneath a retinal venule in the nontapetal fundus. Numerous linear gray "tracks" represent sites of larval migration. Retinal hemorrhage is present in both the tapetal and nontapetal areas.

(Image courtesy of Nancy M. Bromberg, VMD, DACVO.)

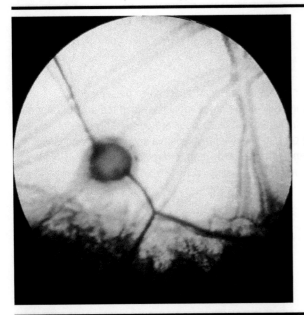

Figure 335
Chorioretinopathy/Ophthalmomyiasis
(2-year-old domestic shorthair)

Missing for 2 days, this cat returned home with a red left eye. A hemorrhagic anterior uveitis prevented evaluation of the posterior segment, but the right eye was normal. Following 1 week of treatment, the anterior uveitis cleared sufficiently to reveal linear, well-demarcated, hyperreflective "tracks" in the tapetal retina. Corresponding tracks appeared light gray within the nontapetal fundus. There were no signs of active chorioretinitis. Although no larvae were observed, the lesions are compatible with subretinal larval migration.

(Image courtesy of B. Keith Collins, DVM, MS, DACVO.)

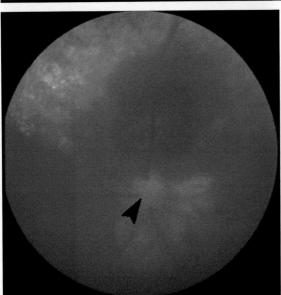

Figure 336
Chorioretinitis/Traumatic
(2.5-year-old Siamese)

This cat was initially examined for eyelid and nictitans lacerations. The anterior chamber was filled with a large blood clot that prevented examination of the fundus. Ten days after treatment for the uveitis, the optic disc (*arrow*) is surrounded by massive subretinal hemorrhage. Resorbing hemorrhage superior to the disc appears darker in color. The overall appearance of the fundus is red because of tapetal hypoplasia and normal lack of pigment within this color-dilute breed.

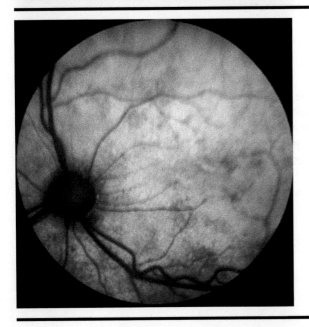

Figure 337
Hypertensive retinopathy
(12-year-old domestic shorthair)

Following a diagnosis of hypertension by the primary veterinarian, this cat was referred for ocular examination. This left eye has subtle focal retinal edema and tapetal discoloration. There was no apparent retinal hemorrhage. The right eye had severe intravitreal hemorrhage and a detached retina.

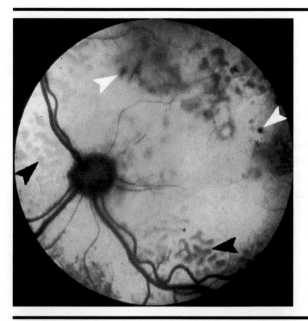

Figure 338
Hypertensive retinopathy/Retinal detachment
(9-year-old domestic longhair)

Presented for evaluation of dark spots on the iris, this cat had a normal pupillary light reflex and functionally normal vision. Both eyes were similarly affected. The dark linear foci (*black arrows*) represent retinal folds caused by edema. The retina to the right of the disc is detached, blurring the detail of the underlying tissue. Focal intraretinal hemorrhages (*white arrows*) are also present. This cat had a blood urea nitrogen (BUN) of 71 mg/dl, a creatinine of 3.1 mg/dl, a systolic blood pressure greater than 300 mm Hg, and generalized cardiomegaly.

(Reproduced from *Veterinary Ocular Pathology: A Comparative Review*. Dubielzig, Ketring, McLellan, Albert. Elsevier Limited, 2010.)

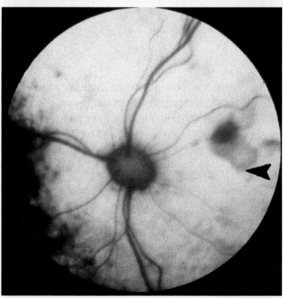

Figure 339
Hypertensive retinopathy
(12-year-old domestic shorthair)

Intraocular hemorrhage had spontaneously resolved prior to this cat's initial evaluation. Mild aqueous flare and slight iris swelling were present bilaterally. Vision and pupillary light reflexes were normal. The tapetum has a mottled appearance due to abnormal pigmentation and diffuse but mild edema. Intraretinal and subretinal hemorrhages are also present (*arrow*). The physical and laboratory findings confirmed hypertension (systolic blood pressure 230 mm Hg) and hyperthyroidism.

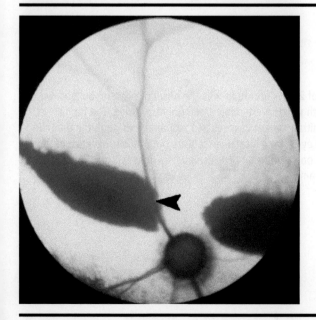

Figure 340
Hypertensive retinopathy
(13-year-old domestic shorthair)

This hypertensive cat had a systolic blood pressure of 260 mm Hg. The left eye is somewhat atypical with only large areas of subretinal hemorrhage. The superior retinal vessel can be seen coursing over the area of hemorrhage (*arrow*).

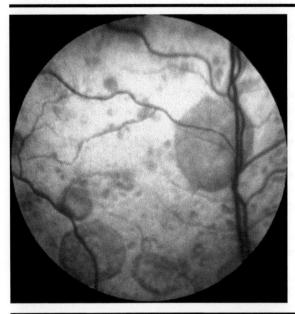

Figure 341
Hypertensive retinopathy
(10-year-old domestic shorthair)

Of a CBC, serum chemistry profile, and routine serologic tests, the only significant abnormality was a mild elevation of BUN in this patient. A subsequent blood pressure measurement documented a mean systolic pressure of 220 mm Hg. Both eyes were similar, with normal vision and normal pupillary reflexes. Multiple rounded foci of edema alter the tapetal reflection. Fluid accumulation is sufficient at some sites to elevate the overlying retina. No retinal hemorrhage was seen.

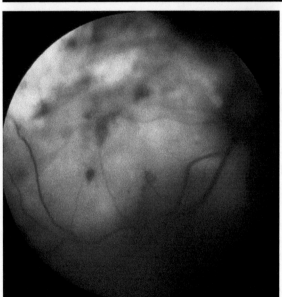

Figure 342
Hypertensive retinopathy/Retinal detachment
(12-year-old domestic shorthair)

This cat was presented for decreased vision of 2 weeks' duration. Mild aqueous flare was noted bilaterally, but pupillary light reflexes were normal. The entire retina is edematous, with an inferior bullous detachment and scattered subretinal hemorrhages. Mild azotemia (BUN 36 mg/dl) accompanied a mean systolic blood pressure of 230 mm Hg.

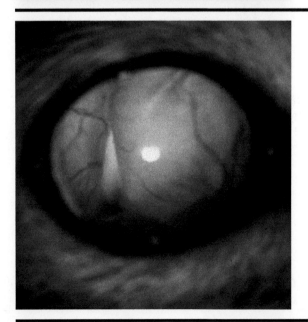

Figure 343
Hypertensive retinopathy/Retinal detachment
(18.5-year-old Somali)

Acute blindness of 2 days' duration was the result of bilateral bullous retinal detachments. Both pupils were dilated and nonresponsive. The retina appears as a semitransparent vascularized membrane through the dilated pupil of the right eye. Some retinal vessels are out of focus because of the detachment. The only abnormal test result was a mean systolic blood pressure of 210 mm Hg.

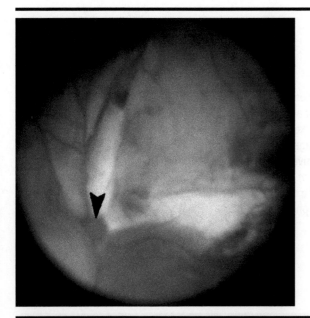

Figure 344
Hypertensive retinopathy/Retinal detachment
(14-year-old domestic longhair)

This cat had a history of progressive vision loss for 2 weeks, resulting in blindness 2 days prior to evaluation. Fundus structures appear small in this photograph, taken through a 28-diopter lens. The optic disc (*arrow*) can be seen at the apex of a large bullous detachment. Intraretinal and subretinal hemorrhages are also present. The only abnormal laboratory or physical finding was a systolic blood pressure of 280 mm Hg.

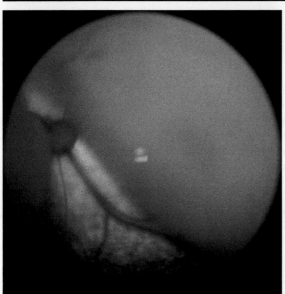

Figure 345
Hypertensive retinopathy/Retinal detachment
(13-year-old domestic shorthair)

This hypertensive cat was referred to determine the likelihood of vision return. At presentation the cat was blind, with fixed, dilated pupils. Large areas of the tapetal fundus appear featureless due to extensive bullous retinal detachment. Only the optic disc and a small diagonal section of edematous retina are recognizable. No hemorrhage was present in either eye. The systolic blood pressure was 260 mm Hg.

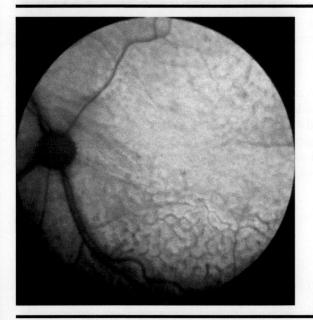

Figure 346
Hypertensive retinopathy/Retinal detachment
(13-year-old domestic shorthair)

This is the same eye of the cat featured in Figure 345 following 1 month of treatment for its hypertension. The pupils are now responsive and the cat is visual. The dark vermiform lesions represent persisting edema in the outer retinal layers, but the bullous detachments have resolved.

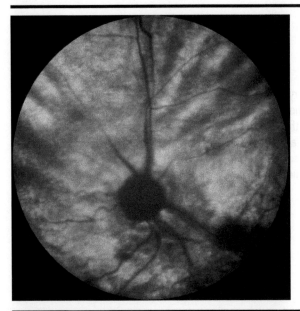

Figure 347
Hypertensive retinopathy/Retinal degeneration
(13-year-old domestic shorthair)

Twenty months prior to examination, this cat was blind with a total bullous retinal detachment and mild intraretinal hemorrhage. Its blood pressure and pupillary light reflexes had returned to normal in response to therapy, and the cat was once again visual. Secondary retinal degeneration is suggested by the hyperreflective tapetum and its furrows of darker coloration that mimic the pattern of the deeper choroidal vessels. The optic disc appears dark because of the neutral density filter used to minimize the tapetal reflectivity for the photograph.

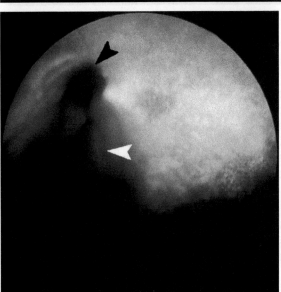

Figure 348
Retinal detachment/Post-traumatic
(4-year-old domestic shorthair)

Examined for decreased vision and a red left eye, this cat had a history of severe head trauma as a kitten. Anterior uveitis and intraocular hemorrhage accounted for the current ocular redness. The right retina hangs from the optic disc (*black arrow*) in an inverted V shape and is no longer attached peripherally at the ora ciliaris. Vessels (*white arrow*) can be seen within the retina, but the adjacent tapetal fundus is notably avascular and hyperreflective.

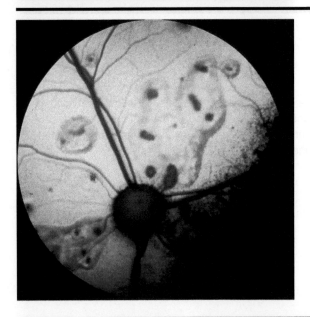

Figure 349
Retinitis/Traumatic
(2-year-old domestic shorthair)

The left globe was proptosed when this cat was hit by a car 24 hours ago. He now appears to be blind in the remaining right eye, the pupil of which is widely dilated and nonresponsive. Multiple deep retinal lesions are scattered throughout the tapetal fundus, with central foci of abnormal pigment surrounded by edema. A few of the lesions appear hyperreflective as the direction of incident light changes.

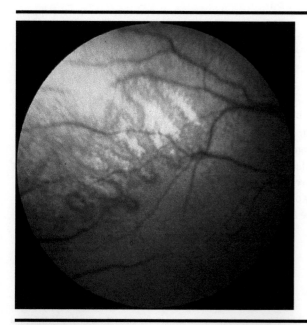

Figure 350
Retinopathy/Traumatic
(4-year-old Siamese)

Anterior uveitis was initially present in the right eye following head trauma. The nasal left fundus appears corrugated, with darkly marginated bands of tapetal hyperreflectivity. This finding is compatible with resolving retinal edema and trauma-induced retinal folds.

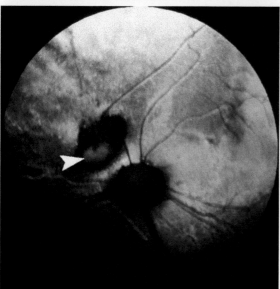

Figure 351
Retinopathy/Post-inflammatory
(6-year-old domestic shorthair)

One year prior to presentation, this cat had been treated for a retrobulbar abscess of the right eye. The owners recently noted pupils of unequal size. The pupil in this eye was dilated with no direct or indirect pupillary light reflexes, while the left reflexes were normal. The optic disc is atrophic. Dorsal retinal vessels are attenuated against the mottled, hyperreflective tapetal background. The sclera (*arrow*) is visible due to loss of overlying choroid and outer retinal layers; surrounding choroidal pigment is hyperplastic. This is a blind eye.

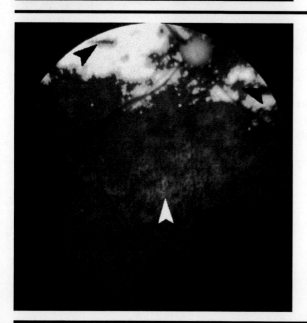

Figure 352
Retinopathy/Post-traumatic
(1.5-year-old domestic shorthair)

This outdoor cat, rarely seen by its owners, was believed to have been hit by a car several months prior to examination. The cat is functionally blind, with dilated and areflexic pupils. The optic disc is subjectively pale and the retinal vessels appear mildly attenuated. Abnormal pigment (*black arrows*) is present at the tapetal-nontapetal junction. Areas of depigmentation interspersed with foci of pigment hypertrophy create a cobblestone appearance (*white arrow*) within the nontapetal fundus. Blindness was attributed to atrophy of the outer retinal layers, a consequence of the cat's initial trauma.

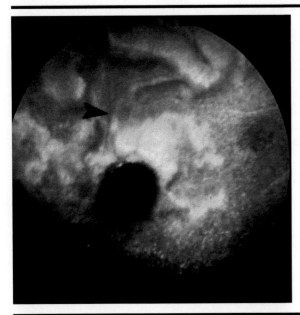

Figure 353
Retinopathy/Idiopathic
(1-year-old domestic shorthair)

The referring veterinarian noticed a mild anisocoria but could appreciate no change in vision. Pupillary light reflexes in the right eye were normal but reflexes in this left eye were sluggish. Few retinal vessels remain (*arrow*). The optic disc is atrophic, although the dark color is primarily an effect of photographic technique. The tapetum is generally hyperreflective, as evident immediately above the dark, circular optic disc. Note that the degree of reflectivity in any one area can vary substantially during the examination, dependent on the angle of incident light. The cause of this retinal atrophy was unknown.

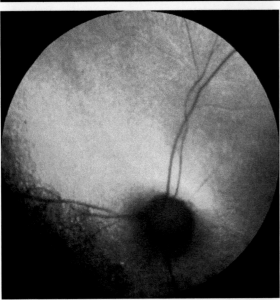

Figure 354
Fluoroquinolone retinopathy
(8-year-old domestic shorthair)

This photograph was taken 6 days after discontinuing a course of enrofloxacin. The cat, now blind, began demonstrating decreased vision on day 4 of treatment. The photograph was taken with a neutral density filter to preserve fundus detail in the face of extreme tapetal hyperreflectivity. As a consequence, the optic disc appears darker than normal. The increased tapetal reflectivity is accompanied by retinal vessel attenuation. A later image of the fundus can be seen in Figure 355.

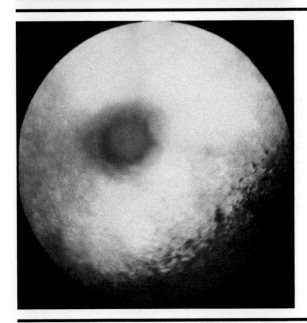

Figure 355
Fluoroquinolone retinopathy
(8-year-old domestic shorthair)

Eight months later, the eye depicted in Figure 354 was reexamined. Even with a neutral density filter, the tapetum appears notably hyperreflective. The retinal vessels are now severely attenuated and difficult to distinguish.

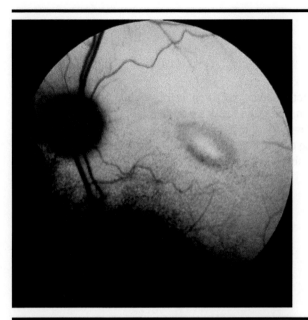

Figure 356
Feline central retinal degeneration
(7.5-year-old Siamese)

As in most cases of feline central retinal degeneration (FCRD), the disorder's bilaterally symmetrical lesions were a coincidental finding. In this left eye, an elliptical area of tapetal hyperreflectivity is evident within the area centralis, the region temporal and superior to the optic disc. The margin of the lesion appears characteristically darker than its reflective center. A neutral density filter causes the normal optic disc to appear unusually dark in color.

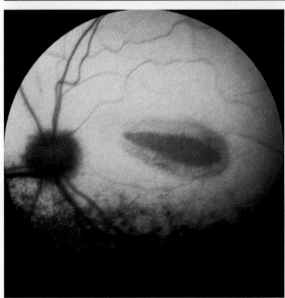

Figure 357
Feline central retinal degeneration
(12-year-old Siamese)

Presented for evaluation of an iris mass in the right eye, this bilateral retinal degeneration was a coincidental finding. The increasing size of the elliptical lesion within the area centralis indicates a more advanced stage of the disorder. The lesion's reflectivity varies as the incidence of the examination beam changes. A slight variation in direction of the light will cause the dark center to appear hyperreflective and its margins to conversely darken, as seen in Figure 356.

(Reproduced from *Veterinary Ocular Pathology: A Comparative Review*. Dubielzig, Ketring, McLellan, Albert. Elsevier Limited, 2010.)

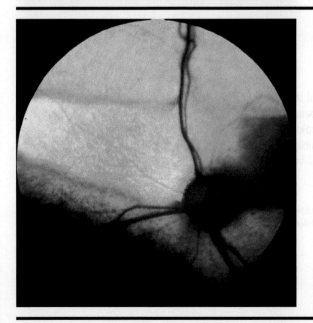

Figure 358
Feline central retinal degeneration
(14-year-old domestic shorthair)

This case was referred for retinal evaluation following a routine physical examination. A large horizontal band of abnormal tapetal reflectivity extends nasally and temporally above the optic disc. As the angle of incident light varies, the appearance of the lesion alternates from light and shiny (left of disc) to dark and dull (right of disc). Although the lesion was bilateral, no vision deficit was detected.

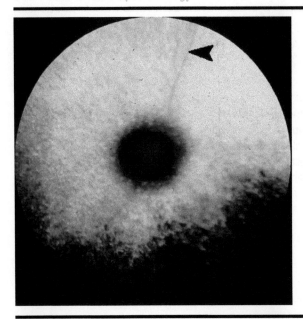

Figure 359
Feline generalized retinal atrophy
(4-month-old domestic shorthair)

The owners had not observed any vision deficit in this kitten until 1 month before examination. The kitten was fed a commercial cat food. Both pupils were dilated, but responded to a bright focal beam. The optic disc is dark because of the use of a neutral density filter. Only one attenuated retinal vessel (*arrow*) persists. The tapetum is brilliantly hyperreflective.

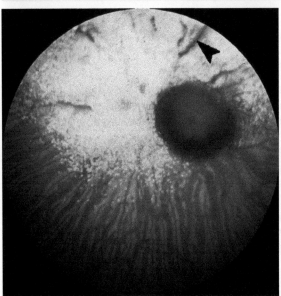

Figure 360
Feline generalized retinal atrophy
(1.5-year-old domestic shorthair)

This cat was examined because of dilated pupils and blindness of 2 weeks' duration. Normal choroidal vessels (*arrow*) are visible within the dorsal fundus because of tapetal hypoplasia and color dilution. The tapetum is hyperreflective, appearing almost white in color. The optic disc is pale, and few retinal vessels can be detected.

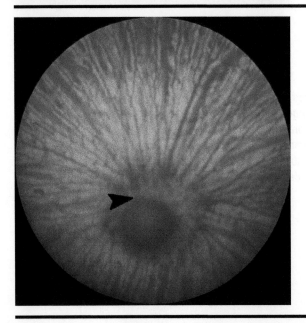

Figure 361
Feline generalized retinal atrophy
(1-year-old domestic shorthair)

The owners noted that the pupils had been dilated for months, but the cat only recently appeared blind. The pupils were responsive only to a bright focal beam. Choroidal vessels and the underlying sclera are normally visible in the atapetal, albinotic white cat. The optic disc is pale. Only a few attenuated retinal vessels can be seen at the superior margin of the disc (*arrow*).

(Reproduced from *Veterinary Ocular Pathology: A Comparative Review*. Dubielzig, Ketring, McLellan, Albert. Elsevier Limited, 2010.)

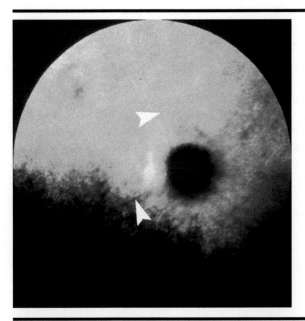

Figure 362
Progressive retinal atrophy
(7-month-old Abyssinian)

Vision had never been normal according to this cat's owners, but function had definitely deteriorated over the last several months. The cat could now see only in very bright light. Both eyes were similarly affected with sluggish pupillary light reflexes. The tapetum is uniformly hyperreflective. The optic disc was pale in appearance, though its color here is altered by use of a neutral density filter. Severely attenuated vessels can be seen extending from the optic disc (*arrows*).

(Reproduced from *Veterinary Ocular Pathology: A Comparative Review*. Dubielzig, Ketring, McLellan, Albert. Elsevier Limited, 2010.)

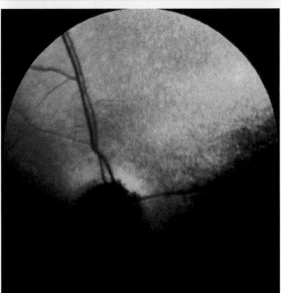

Figure 363
Progressive retinal atrophy
(6-year-old Abyssinian)

Vision had been equally poor in both bright and dim light for about 1 year. The pupillary light reflexes were sluggish but present in both eyes. Attempts at visual testing were unrewarding because of the cat's uncooperative nature. All retinal vessels are attenuated and the tapetum is generally hyperreflective. The only abnormality in the nontapetal area was the subjective attenuation of retinal vessels. The optic disc appears dark due to the neutral density filter used for photography.

(Reproduced from *Veterinary Ocular Pathology: A Comparative Review*. Dubielzig, Ketring, McLellan, Albert. Elsevier Limited, 2010.)

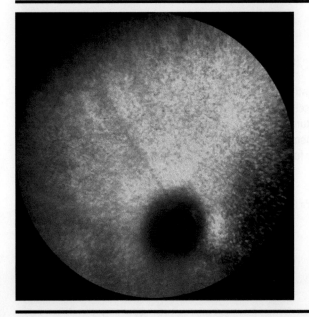

Figure 364
Progressive retinal atrophy
(3-year-old Tonkinese)

Owners had noticed a decrease in night vision for several months. The dilated pupils responded poorly to bright light. Clinically the optic disc appeared pale; a neutral density filter darkens the disc in the image. The tapetum still appears hyperreflective, even with the dampening effect of the filter. Retinal vessels are severely attenuated.

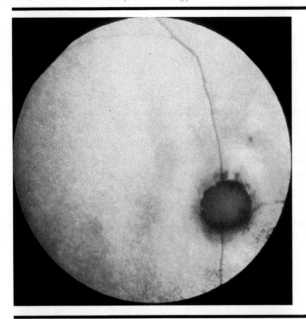

Figure 365
Progressive retinal atrophy
(3-year-old Burmese)

The owners reported gradual vision loss in their cat, which could now see only in bright light. They also noted in the last 6 months that the eyes "glowed." The pupillary light reflexes, although present, were very sluggish. This photograph, taken with a neutral density filter, shows severely attenuated retinal vessels and diffuse tapetal hyperreflectivity. The optic disc is pale, but appears darker in the photograph because of use of the filter.

(Reproduced from *Veterinary Ocular Pathology: A Comparative Review*. Dubielzig, Ketring, McLellan, Albert. Elsevier Limited, 2010.)

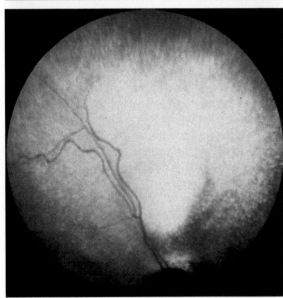

Figure 366
Progressive retinal atrophy
(14-year-old Siamese)

The owners recently noted dilated pupils and cloudy lenses, but acknowledged that vision had been poor for several years. The pupils were dilated and poorly responsive to a bright focal beam. Lenticular nuclear sclerosis was present in both eyes, but no cataract formation was observed. The tapetum is markedly hyperreflective. The retinal vessels are reduced in number, caliber, and degree of branching.

(Reproduced from *Veterinary Ocular Pathology: A Comparative Review*. Dubielzig, Ketring, McLellan, Albert. Elsevier Limited, 2010.)

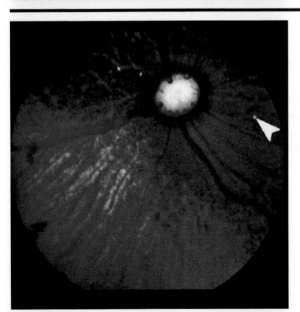

Figure 367
Chediak–Higashi syndrome
(9-month-old Persian)

Coat and iris coloration in this cat were typical of the disease. Only small islands of tapetal cells (*arrow*) remain following tapetal degeneration. Choroidal vasculature is visible because of the decreased amount of melanin in the retinal pigmented epithelium. This depigmentation may progress to a complete albinotic fundus. This cat's anterior segment is illustrated in Figure 173.

(Image courtesy of Linda L. Collier, DVM, PhD, DACVO.)

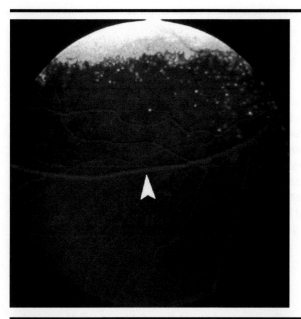

Figure 368
Lipemia retinalis
(5.5-year-old domestic shorthair)

This cat was being treated with oral corticosteroids on alternate days to control an eosinophilic gastritis. She was presented for evaluation of a mild unilateral ocular discharge. The tapetal retina appeared entirely normal. The retinal vessels are cream colored against the pigmented background of the nontapetal fundus. As the vessels decrease in caliber distal to the optic disc (*arrow*), the cream color is more remarkable. The lipid cleared when the corticosteroids were temporarily discontinued.

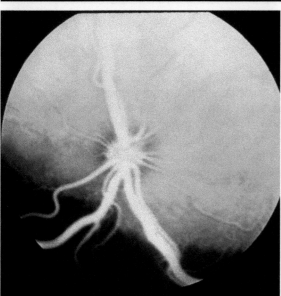

Figure 369
Lipemia retinalis
(domestic shorthair kitten)

This kitten had experimentally induced diabetes mellitus. Even the retinal vessels within the tapetal fundus appear cream colored because of the severity of the associated hyperlipidemia.

(Image courtesy of C. Sue West, DVM, DACVO.)

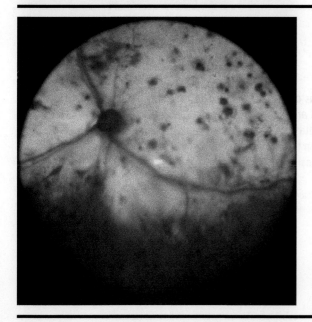

Figure 370
Retinitis/Plasma cell tumor
(13-year-old Himalayan)

Presented to the referring veterinarian for anorexia and lethargy, this cat had widespread bilateral intraretinal hemorrhages throughout the fundus. The small circular ("dot") shape is typical of hemorrhage constrained by the compact nature of the superficial retina. Abnormal laboratory findings included a severe hyperproteinemia, hypergammaglobulinemia, a moderate anemia and severe thrombocytopenia. A fine-needle aspirate of the liver provided the final diagnosis.

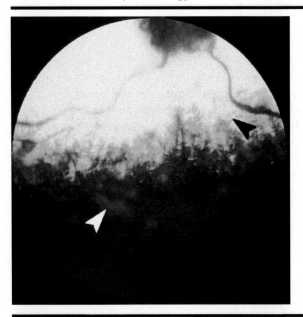

Figure 371
Retinitis/Lymphoma
(2-year-old domestic shorthair)

Lethargy, ataxia, and blindness were present for 1 week in this cat. The pupils were dilated and nonresponsive. Ocular lesions were bilateral and restricted to the fundus. The wide linear gray areas seen in the nontapetal fundus (*white arrow*) are caused by edema in the outer layers of the retina. The associated vessels are not elevated. The orange bands (*black arrow*) represent the same condition in the tapetal region. The optic nerve involvement is better depicted in Figure 391. The feline leukemia virus test was negative, but large abnormal lymphocytes were found in the optic nerve meninges, leading to the diagnosis of lymphoma.

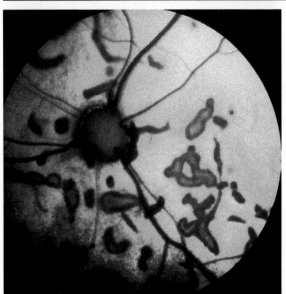

Figure 372
Retinitis/Lymphoma
(15-month-old domestic shorthair)

At 10 months of age, the left eye of this cat was enucleated due to a retrobulbar mass diagnosed as lymphoma. In spite of ongoing therapy, he became acutely blind in the remaining right eye. The pupil was dilated and nonresponsive. Multiple vermiform lesions with pink centers and pigmented margins are scattered throughout the tapetal fundus. These are located in the deeper layers of the retina, since the course of overlying vessels is unaltered.

(Reproduced from *Veterinary Ocular Pathology: A Comparative Review*. Dubielzig, Ketring, McLellan, Albert. Elsevier Limited, 2010.)

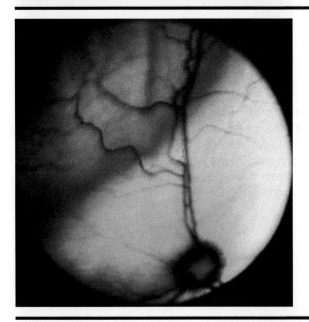

Figure 373
Retrobulbar lymphoma
(7-year-old domestic shorthair)

This is the fundus of the cat in Figure 26, captured through a 28-diopter lens. The dark tapetal area extending from the 8-o'clock to 1-o'clock position is due to the indentation of the globe by a retrobulbar tumor. As the eye moved in relation to the mass, the area of elevation would change. The histologic diagnosis was retrobulbar lymphoma.

(Reproduced from *Veterinary Ocular Pathology: A Comparative Review*. Dubielzig, Ketring, McLellan, Albert. Elsevier Limited, 2010.)

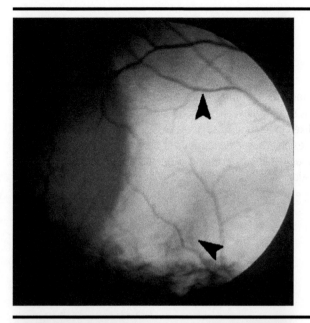

Figure 374
Retinal elevation/Retrobulbar neoplasia
(3-year-old domestic shorthair)

A firm mass was palpable between the nictitans and orbital rim of the cat first described in Figure 22. The posterior scleral surface is distorted by a retrobulbar mass, creating a dark shadow in the nasal fundus (left side of photograph). The tapetum appears less reflective at adjacent retinal elevations (*arrows*). Shadows would change position relative to the optic disc as the globe moved over the retrobulbar mass. An undifferentiated sarcoma was diagnosed by a fine-needle aspirate of the tumor.

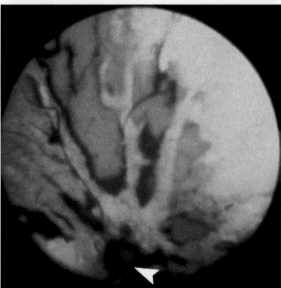

Figure 375
Retinal atrophy/Metastatic intestinal adenocarcinoma
(14-year-old domestic shorthair)

This cat was presented with anorexia, weight loss, ataxia, and decreased vision; its pupils were dilated and nonresponsive. The extent of the fundic abnormality is apparent in the wide field provided by the 28-diopter lens. The optic disc is located at the ventral margin of the field (*white arrow*). The normal tapetal fundus has been supplanted by well-demarcated gray infiltrates, pigment, hyperreflectivity, and attenuated retinal vessels. On histopathology, tumor cells were identified in the small intestine, spleen, optic nerve meninges, and retinal and choroidal vessels.

(Reproduced from *Veterinary Ocular Pathology: A Comparative Review*. Dubielzig, Ketring, McLellan, Albert. Elsevier Limited, 2010.)

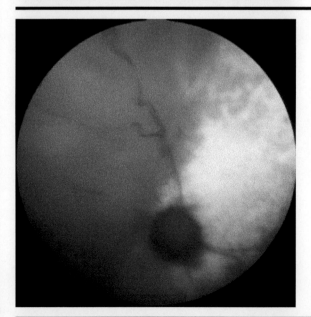

Figure 376
Chorioretinitis/Metastatic adenocarcinoma
(12-year-old domestic shorthair)

The patient's presenting complaints included a red right eye and a dilated, sluggish pupil in this left eye. A large gray mass within the retina and choroid obscures the tapetal reflection. In some areas, the neoplasm breaches the retinal surface and obscures the retinal vessels. The primary site of this tumor was not identified.

(Reproduced from *Veterinary Ocular Pathology: A Comparative Review*. Dubielzig, Ketring, McLellan, Albert. Elsevier Limited, 2010.)

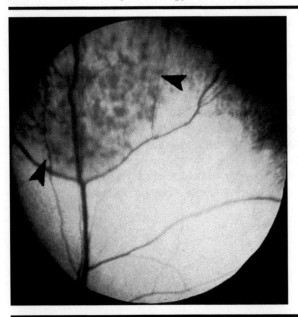

Figure 377
Retinal detachment/Metastatic hemangiosarcoma
(1.5-year-old Siamese)

This is the right superior temporal retina of the cat in Figure 243. A red, mottled infiltrate is slightly elevated and obscures the tapetum (*arrows*). The lesion remained fixed in relation to adjacent vessels as the globe moved, in contrast to those lesions caused by retrobulbar masses (see Figure 374). Metastatic choroidal hemangiosarcoma was diagnosed on histopathology following enucleation.

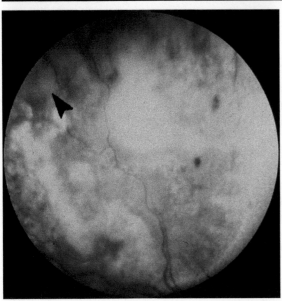

Figure 378
Chorioretinitis/Metastatic adenocarcinoma
(7-year-old domestic shorthair)

A complaint of lameness and erosions of all four paws preceded the onset of anisocoria. Mild aqueous flare was present bilaterally. A well-demarcated zone of altered tapetal reflectivity occupies the dorsonasal quadrant of the left fundus. Subretinal exudates (*arrow*) elevate the retina. Focal hemorrhages are seen near the margin of the lesion. Histopathology of the digits and eye was compatible with adenocarcinoma of sweat gland origin.

SECTION XII

Optic Nerve

Atlas of Feline Ophthalmology. Second Edition. Kerry L. Ketring and Mary Belle Glaze.
© 2012 John Wiley & Sons, Inc. Published 2012 by John Wiley & Sons, Inc.

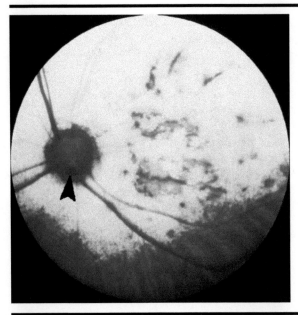

Figure 379
Optic disc coloboma
(4-year-old Siamese)

This cat was presented for an unrelated conjunctivitis. The red streaks are normal choroidal vessels seen in areas of tapetal hypoplasia. A small dark area (*arrow*) at the edge of the disc represents a gap or fissure in the ocular tissue known as a coloboma.

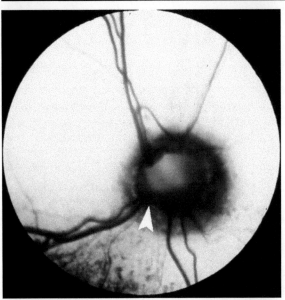

Figure 380
Optic disc coloboma
(8-month-old American shorthair)

To explain the loss of vision in the right eye, the referring veterinarian theorized that unobserved trauma had caused a retinal detachment in this cat at 1 month of age. The cat did appear blind in the right eye. Rapid rotary nystagmus was present bilaterally, but pupillary light reflexes were normal in the left eye. A dark pigmented ring surrounds the left optic disc. The retinal vessels (*arrows*) disappear from view as they cross the rim of a large coloboma. The size of the defect, its featureless character, and its gray color distinguish this circular congenital defect from the normal optic disc. The right fundus appears in Figure 383.

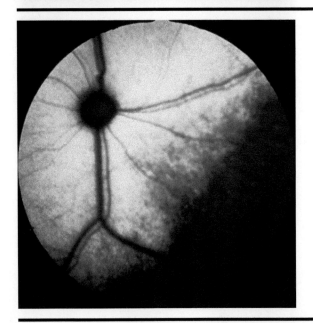

Figure 381
Optic disc hypoplasia
(1.5-year-old Himalayan)

Presented for evaluation of chronic conjunctivitis, this cat had normal pupillary light responses and vision in both eyes. Subjectively, the optic disc appears smaller than normal. This is especially evident when the disc size is compared to the retinal vein. Both eyes were similarly affected. A neutral density filter accounts for the extreme darkness of the disc.

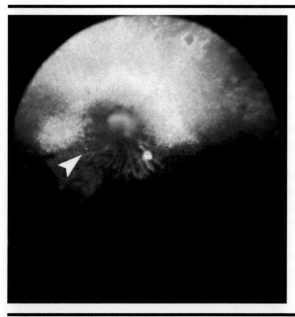

Figure 382
Optic disc aplasia
(9-month-old domestic shorthair)

This blind kitten has had dilated, areflexic pupils since birth. He recently developed an upper respiratory infection that responded to supportive treatment. Although presented for evaluation of entropion, the most remarkable lesions were found within the fundus of both eyes. This photograph, taken through a 28-diopter lens, shows severe tapetal hyperreflectivity with no detectable retinal vessels. In the area that should contain the optic disc, branching white striae (*arrow*) are evident overlying the tapetum. A gray amorphous mass supplants the optic disc. There were no signs of previous or active inflammation or infection in any part of the eye. The opposite fundus was also hyperreflective and devoid of retinal vessels.

(Reproduced from *Veterinary Ocular Pathology: A Comparative Review*. Dubielzig, Ketring, McLellan, Albert. Elsevier Limited, 2010.)

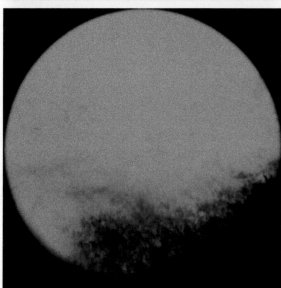

Figure 383
Optic disc aplasia
(8-month-old American shorthair)

The photograph, taken through a 28-diopter lens, is of the right fundus of the cat in Figure 380. The photograph shows the area that should contain the optic disc. The tapetum is hyperreflective. Neither the retinal vessels nor any remnants of the optic disc could be found on ophthalmoscopic examination.

(Reproduced from *Veterinary Ocular Pathology: A Comparative Review*. Dubielzig, Ketring, McLellan, Albert. Elsevier Limited, 2010.)

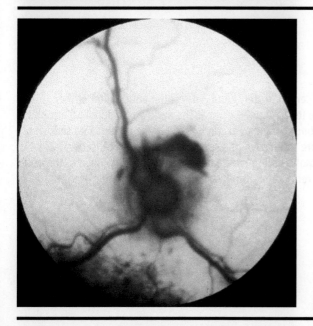

Figure 384
Optic neuritis/Cryptococcosis
(2-year-old domestic shorthair)

This cat had been diagnosed with cryptococcal meningitis on the basis of a cerebrospinal fluid tap. In the last several days, vision had deteriorated. The anterior segment, including pupillary light reflexes, was normal. The cat followed cotton balls, but vision was subjectively poor. Optic disc abnormalities were comparable bilaterally. The dark color around the optic disc is due to hemorrhage in the nerve fiber layer. Subretinal edema and hemorrhage have elevated the peripapillary retina, obscuring detail of the swollen optic disc.

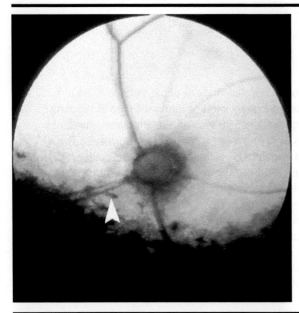

Figure 385
Optic nerve atrophy/Toxoplasmosis
(4-year-old domestic longhair)

Weight loss was noted in this cat for about 5 months prior to the onset of blindness 5 days ago. Both pupils were fixed and dilated. Optic nerve atrophy is suggested by the gray optic disc and the exaggerated sieve-like appearance of the lamina cribrosa. Abnormal tapetal pigment is present (*arrow*). Two areas of focal retinal edema were noted but are not visible in this photograph. Laboratory tests were unremarkable and included negative FIV and FeLV results. The owners elected euthanasia. Histopathologic examination showed focal areas of retinal pigment epithelial cells within the sensory retina. Lymphocytes and plasma cells were found infiltrating both optic nerves. Two spherical cysts containing numerous elongated organisms suggestive of *Toxoplasma* were found in one optic nerve. A titer for toxoplasmosis was not available.

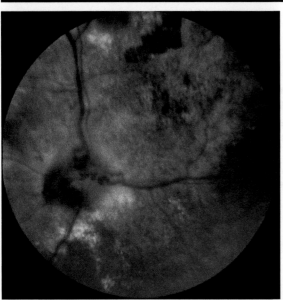

Figure 386
Optic nerve atrophy/Histoplasmosis
(3-year-old domestic shorthair)

Despite resolution of systemic signs following treatment for histoplasmosis, this patient's optic nerve and retina degenerated as a consequence of the prolonged posterior segment inflammation. The optic disc is darkly pigmented, with an abnormally tortuous vessel at its dorsal margin. Pigment of varying density replaces the tapetum. The pale area near the optic disc represents exposed sclera.

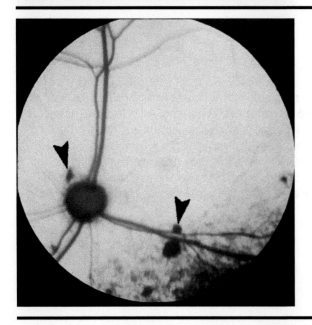

Figure 387
Optic nerve/Retinal atrophy
(4-year-old domestic shorthair)

This cat was presented acutely blind 2 days after enucleation of the contralateral eye for a ruptured cornea. The optic disc is dark and atrophic. Focal areas of abnormal pigment can be seen in the tapetal area (*arrows*). These findings are suggestive of a surgical complication caused by excessive traction on the globe during enucleation. The resulting damage to the optic chiasm leads to retrograde atrophy of the contralateral optic nerve.

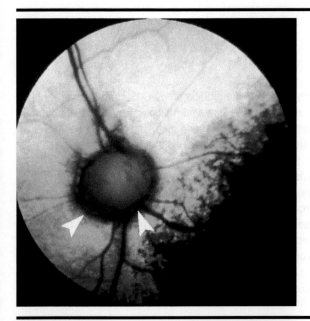

Figure 388
Optic nerve atrophy/Glaucoma
(2-year-old domestic shorthair)

This cat was presented for evaluation of a cloudy left cornea resulting from an anterior lens luxation (see Figure 288). The anterior chambers were deep in both eyes, with positive pupillary light reflexes and iridodonesis. The lens in the right eye was subluxated. The intraocular pressure was 34 mm Hg in the right eye and 20 mm Hg in the left. Both globes were mildly buphthalmic. The optic disc in the right eye appears larger than normal because of glaucomatous cupping. The cupping is more remarkable temporally and inferiorly (*arrows*), where the vessels can be seen disappearing over the rim of the cup.

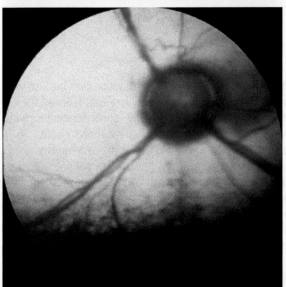

Figure 389
Optic nerve atrophy/Glaucoma
(10-year-old domestic shorthair)

A progressive darkening of the iris and enlargement of the left globe over the past 2 years preceded this cat's examination. The iris was uniformly thickened and heavily pigmented. The pupil was dilated and pupillary light reflexes were negative. Pigment was present on the anterior lens capsule. The intraocular pressure was greater than 60 mm Hg. The optic disc is uniformly cupped and atrophic, giving the appearance of an enlarged disc. Peripapillary retinal atrophy is present, but the remaining retina appears normal. Histopathology confirmed an iris melanoma and atrophy of the optic nerve.

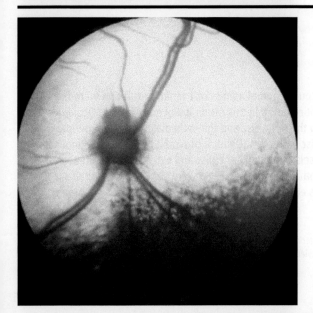

Figure 390
Optic nerve glioma
(15-year-old domestic shorthair)

During evaluation of a diffuse iris mass in the opposite eye, a discrete gray nodule was noted on and adjacent to the right optic disc. The intraretinal mass surrounds nearby retinal vessels. Vision and pupillary light reflexes were normal. The clinical appearance was suggestive of a glioma, although there was no opportunity for histopathological confirmation of that diagnosis.

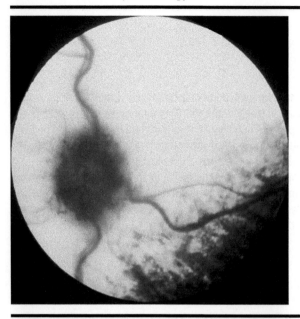

Figure 391
Optic neuritis/Lymphoma
(2-year-old domestic shorthair)

A history of lethargy, ataxia, and blindness of 1 week's duration were complaints voiced at this cat's examination. All laboratory tests were normal, including a negative test for feline leukemia virus. The pupillary light reflexes were absent in both eyes. All lesions were bilateral and limited to the posterior segment. Mild retinal edema is present. The retinal vessels, especially the arterioles, are tortuous and extend over the swollen optic disc. There is also neovascularization of the disc and surrounding retina. Faint areas of hemorrhage are present within the nerve fiber layer. Other fundus lesions are depicted in Figure 371. A diagnosis of lymphoma was based on histopathologic evidence of large neoplastic lymphocytes that infiltrated the meninges of both optic nerves.

(Reproduced from *Veterinary Ocular Pathology: A Comparative Review*. Dubielzig, Ketring, McLellan, Albert. Elsevier Limited, 2010.)

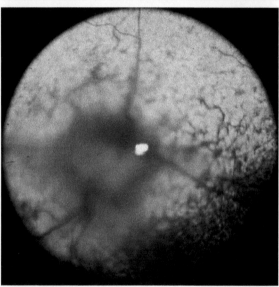

Figure 392
Optic neuritis/Lymphoma
(10-year-old domestic shorthair)

This cat was presented for a progressive decrease in vision over the last month. The cat was functionally blind with no pupillary light reflexes. The right eye had a severe anterior uveitis and a massive retinal detachment with intraretinal hemorrhage. This photograph of the left eye shows a pale, ill-defined mass overlying the optic disc, accompanied by peripapillary retinal edema. Intraretinal hemorrhage is also present. The peripheral retina was edematous and a large temporal bullous detachment was present. Histopathology documented neoplastic cells, primarily within the uveal tract. The optic nerve head contained clusters of neoplastic cells, but the clinical picture was most likely explained by secondary necrosis with an inflammatory cell infiltrate.

(Reproduced from *Veterinary Ocular Pathology: A Comparative Review*. Dubielzig, Ketring, McLellan, Albert. Elsevier Limited, 2010.)

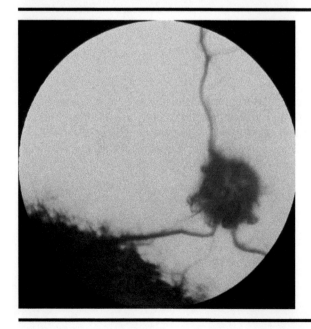

Figure 393
Optic neuritis/Meningioma
(8-year-old domestic shorthair)

Dilated, areflexic pupils and blindness of 1 month's duration were the only clinical abnormalities noted in this cat on initial examination. Ocular lesions were restricted to the optic disc and the immediately adjacent peripapillary area. The optic disc is swollen. Detail is obscured by adjacent retinal edema and tortuous vessels that overlie the disc and extend into the immediate peripapillary retina. Three weeks later, the cat started circling, had several seizures, and was euthanatized. Meningioma was the histopathologic diagnosis.

(Reproduced from *Veterinary Ocular Pathology: A Comparative Review*. Dubielzig, Ketring, McLellan, Albert. Elsevier Limited, 2010.)

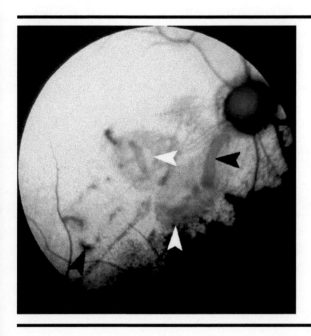

Figure 394
Meningioma
(9-year-old domestic shorthair)

The left eye of this cat had been enucleated 4 months prior to this examination because of blindness and an unresponsive corneal ulcer. Histopathology of the enucleated globe revealed a nonspecific endophthalmitis. The cat was now blind in the remaining eye and had several episodes of head tilt, ataxia, and seizures. The optic disc is light gray and atrophic. Linear areas of abnormal pigmentation are present temporal to the optic disc (*black arrows*). Focal retinal elevations (*white arrows*) are also present. The diagnosis of meningioma was based on histopathologic examination of the optic nerve following euthanasia.

Bibliography

ORBIT
Inflammatory/Infectious Disease

Bernays ME, Peiffer RL: Ocular infections with dematiaceous fungi in two cats and a dog. *J Am Vet Med Assoc* 213: 507–509, 1998.

Bissonnette KW, Sharp NJ, Dykstra MH, et al: Nasal and retrobulbar mass in a cat caused by *Pythium insidiosum*. *J Med Vet Mycol* 29: 39–44, 1991.

Busse C, Dennis R, Platt SR: Suspected sphenoid bone osteomyelitis causing visual impairment in two dogs and one cat. *Vet Ophthalmol* 12: 71–77, 2009.

Dziezyc J, Barton CL, Santos A: Exophthalmia in a cat caused by an eosinophilic infiltrate. *Prog Vet Comp Ophthalmol* 2: 91–93, 1992.

Halenda RM, Reed AL: Fungal sinusitis and retrobulbar myofascitis in a cat. *Vet Radiol Ultrasound* 38: 208–210, 1997.

Lybaert P, Delbecke I, Cohen-Solal A: Diagnosis and management of a wooden foreign body in the orbit of a cat. *J Feline Med Surg* 11: 219–221, 2009.

Peiffer RL, Belkin PV, Janke BH: Orbital cellulitis, sinusitis, and pneumonitis caused by *Penicillium* spp in a cat. *J Am Vet Med Assoc* 176: 449–451, 1980.

Ramsey DT, Marretta SM, Hamor RE, et al: Ophthalmic manifestations and complications of dental disease in dogs and cats. *J Am Anim Hosp Assoc* 32: 215–224, 1996.

Smith MM, Smith EM, La Croix N, et al: Orbital penetration associated with tooth extraction. *J Vet Dent* 20: 8–17, 2003.

Tovar MC, Huguet E, Gomezi MA: Orbital cellulitis and intraocular abscess caused by migrating grass in a cat. *Vet Ophthalmol* 8: 353–356, 2005.

Van der Woerdt A: Orbital inflammatory disease and pseudotumor in dogs and cats. *Vet Clin North Am Small Anim Pract* 38: 389–401, 2008.

Wang AL, Ledbetter EC, Kern TJ: Orbital abscess bacterial isolates and in vitro antimicrobial susceptibility patterns in dogs and cats. *Vet Ophthalmol* 12: 91–96, 2009.

Wolfer J, Grahn B: Orbital emphysema from frontal sinus penetration in a cat. *Can Vet J* 36: 186–187, 1995.

Aspergillosis

Barachetti L, Mortellaro CM, Giancamillo M, et al: Bilateral orbital and nasal aspergillosis in a cat. *Vet Ophthalmol* 12: 176–182, 2009.

Barrs VR, Beatty JA, Lingard AE, et al: Feline sino-orbital aspergillosis: An emerging clinical syndrome. *Aust Vet J* 85: N23, 2007

Giordano C, Gianella P, Bo S, et al: Invasive mould infections of the naso-orbital region of cats: A case involving *Aspergillus fumigates* and an aetiological review. *J Feline Med Surg* 12: 714–723, 2010.

Hamilton HL, Whitely RD, McLaughlin SA: Exophthalmos secondary to aspergillosis in a cat. *J Am Anim Hosp Assoc* 36: 343–347, 2000.

McLellan GJ, Aquino SM, Mason DR, et al: Use of posaconazole in the management of invasive orbital aspergillosis in a cat. *J Am Anim Hosp Assoc* 42: 302–307, 2006.

Smith LN, Hoffman SB: A case series of unilateral orbital aspergillosis in three cats and treatment with voriconazole. *Vet Ophthalmol* 13: 190–203, 2010.

Wilkinson GT, Sutton RH, Grono LR: *Aspergillus* spp infection associated with orbital cellulitis and sinusitis in a cat. *J Small Anim Pract* 23: 127–131, 1982.

Neoplasia

Attali-Soussay K, Jegou J-P, Clerc B: Retrobulbar tumors in dogs and cats: 25 cases. *Vet Ophthalmol* 4: 19–27, 2001.

Court EA, Watson AD, Peaston AE: Retrospective study of 60 cases of feline lymphosarcoma. *Austr Vet J* 75: 424–427, 1997.

Foley RH: Zygomatic osteoma in a cat. *Feline Pract* 21: 26–28, 1993.

Gilger BC, McLaughlin SA, Whitley RD, et al: Orbital neoplasms in cats: 21 cases (1974–1990). *J Am Vet Med Assoc* 201: 1083–1086, 1992.

Groskopf BS, Dubielzig RR, Beaumont SL: Orbital extraskeletal osteosarcoma following enucleation in a cat: A case report. *Vet Ophthalmol* 13: 179–183, 2010.

Hartmann A: Feline exophthalmia. *Vet Forum* 4: 33–37, 2005.

Knecht CD, Greene JA: Osteoma of the zygomatic arch in a cat. *J Am Vet Med Assoc* 171: 1077–1078, 1977.

McCalla TL, Moore CP: Exophthalmos in dogs and cats. Part I. Anatomic and diagnostic considerations. *Compend Contin Educ Pract Vet* 11: 784–792, 1989.

McCalla TL, Moore CP: Exophthalmos in dogs and cats. Part II. *Compend Contin Educ Pract Vet* 11: 911–926, 1989.

Negrin A, Bernardini M, Diana A, et al: Giant cell osteosarcoma in the calvarium of a cat. *Vet Pathol* 43: 179–182, 2006.

Peiffer RL, Spencer C, Popp JA: Nasal squamous cell carcinoma with periocular extension and metastasis in a cat. *Feline Pract* 8: 43–46, 1978.

Pentlarge VW, Powell-Johnson G, Martin CL, et al: Orbital neoplasia with enophthalmos in a cat. *J Am Vet Med Assoc* 195: 1249–1251, 1989.

Ward DA, McEntee MF, Weddle DL: Orbital plasmacytoma in a cat. *J Small Anim Pract* 38: 576–578, 1997.

Wolfer J, Grahn B: Diagnostic ophthalmology. Amelanotic melanoma in an 8-year-old cat. *Can Vet J* 36: 518–519, 1995.

Wray JD, Doust RT, McConnell F: Retrobulbar teratoma causing exophthalmos in a cat. *J Feline Med Surg* 10: 175–180, 2008.

Proptosis

Gilger BC, Hamilton HL, Wilkie DA, et al: Traumatic ocular proptoses in dogs and cats: 84 cases (1980–1993). *J Am Anim Hosp Assoc* 206: 1186–1190, 1995.

Pseudotumor

Billson FM, Miller-Michau T, Mould JRB, et al: Idiopathic sclerosing orbital pseudotumor in seven cats. *Vet Ophthalmol* 9: 45–51, 2006.

Miller SA, van der Woerdt S, Bartick TE: Retrobulbar pseudotumor of the orbit in a cat. *J Am Vet Med Assoc* 216: 356–358, 2000.

Strabismus

Alekseenko SV, Shkorbatova PY, Toporova SN: Interhemisphere connections of the visual cortex in cats with bilateral strabismus. *Neurosci Behav Physiol* 36: 1015–1019, 2006.

Buchtel HA, Berlucchi G, Mascetti GG: Behavioural and electrophysiological analysis of strabismus in cats: modern context. *Exp Brain Res* 192: 359–367, 2009.

Johnson BW: Congenitally abnormal visual pathways of Siamese cats. *Compend Contin Educ Vet* 13: 374–378, 1991.

Schmidt KE, Singer W, Galuske RAW: Processing deficits in primary visual cortex of amblyopic cats. *J Neurophysiol* 91: 1661–1671, 2004.

Miscellaneous

Armour MD, Broome M, Dell 'Anna G, et al: A review of orbital and intracranial magnetic resonance imaging in 79 canine and 13 feline patients (2004-2010). *Vet Ophthalmol* 14: 215–226, 2011.

Cho J: Surgery of the globe and orbit. *Top Comp Anim Med* 23: 23–37, 2008.

Crotti A: Orbital fat prolapse in cats: Two clinical cases. *Proc Ann Mtg Eur Coll Vet Ophthalmol* 2004, p 113.

Dennis R: Use of magnetic resonance imaging for the investigation of orbital disease in small animals. *J Small Anim Pract* 41: 145–155, 2000.

Pooya HA, Seguin B, Tucker RL, et al: Magnetic resonance imaging in small animal medicine: clinical applications. *Compend Contin Educ Vet* 26: 292–302, 2004.

Morgan RV: Ultrasonography of retrobulbar diseases of the dog and cat. *J Am Anim Hosp Assoc* 25: 393–399, 1989.

Nasisse MP, van Ee RT, Munger RJ, et al: Use of methyl methacrylate orbital prostheses in dogs and cats: 78 cases (1980–1986). *J Am Vet Med Assoc* 192: 539–542, 1988.

Ramsey DT, Gerding PA, Losonsky JM, et al: Comparative value of diagnostic imaging techniques in a cat with exophthalmos. *Vet Comp Ophthalmol* 4: 198–202, 1994.

Stiles J, Townsend W, et al: Use of a caudal auricular axial pattern flap in three cats and one dog following orbital exenteration. *Vet Ophthalmol* 6: 121–126, 2003.

Wolfer J, Grahn B: Diagnostic ophthalmology. *Orbital emphysema. Can Vet J* 36: 186–187, 1995.

EYELID

Eyelid Agenesis

Bellhorn RW, Barnett KC, Kendkin P: Ocular colobomas in domestic cats. *J Am Vet Med Assoc* 159: 1015–1021, 1971.

Blogg JR: Agenesis of the feline upper eyelid. *Feline Pract* 15: 31–35, 1985.

Dziezyc J, Millichamp NJ: Surgical correction of eyelid agenesis in a cat. *J Am Anim Hosp Assoc* 25: 513–516, 1989.

Esson D: A modification of the Mustardé technique for the surgical repair of a large feline eyelid coloboma. *Vet Ophthalmol* 4: 159–160, 2001.

Koch SA: Congenital ophthalmic abnormalities in the Burmese cat. *J Am Vet Med Assoc* 174: 90–91, 1979.

Martin CL, Stiles J, Willis M: Feline colobomatous syndrome. *Vet Comp Ophthalmol* 7: 39–43, 1997.

Munger RJ, Gourley IM: Cross lid flap for repair of large upper eyelid defects. *J Am Vet Med Assoc* 178: 45–48, 1981.

Roberts SR, Bistner SI: Surgical correction of eyelid agenesis. *Mod Vet Pract* 49: 40–43, 1968.

Whittaker CJG, Wilkie DA, Simpson DJ, et al: Lip commissure to eyelid transposition for repair of feline eyelid agenesis. *Vet Ophthalmol* 13: 173–178, 2010.

Wolfer JC: Correction of eyelid coloboma in four cats using subdermal collagen and a modified Stades technique. *Vet Ophthalmol* 5: 269–272, 2002.

Entropion

Read RA, Broun HC: Entropion correction in dogs and cats using a combination Hotz-Celsus and lateral eyelid wedge resection: Results in 311 eyes. *Vet Ophthalmol* 10: 6–11, 2007.

van der Woerdt A: Adnexal surgery in dogs and cats. *Vet Ophthalmol* 7: 284–290, 2004.

Weiss CW: Feline entropion. *Fel Pract* 10: 38–40, 1980.

Willliams DL, Kim J-Y: Feline entropion: a case series of 50 affected animals (2003–2008). *Vet Ophthalmol* 12: 221–226, 2009.

Ectopic Cilia

Hacker DV: Ectopic cilia in a Siamese cat. *Comp Anim Pract* 19: 29–31, 1989.

Blepharitis

Barnes JC, Stanley O, Craig TM: Diffuse cutaneous leishmaniasis in a cat. *J Am Vet Med Assoc* 202: 416–418, 1993.

Bond R, Curtis CF, Ferguson EA, et al: An idiopathic facial dermatitis of Persian cats. *Vet Dermatol* 11: 35–41, 2000.

Chung T-H, Ryu M-H, Kim D-Y, et al: Topical tacrolimus (FK506) for the treatment of feline idiopathic facial dermatitis. *Aust Vet J* 87: 417–420, 2009.

Espinolaz MB, Lilenbaum W: Prevalence of bacteria in the conjunctival sac and on the eyelid margin of clinically normal cats. *J Small Anim Pract* 37: 364–366, 1996.

Flecknell PA, Orr CM, Wright AL, et al: Skin ulceration associated with herpesvirus infection in cats. *Vet Rec* 104: 313–315, 1979.

Friberg C: Feline facial dermatoses. *Vet Clin North Am Small Anim Pract* 36: 115–140, 2006.

Hargis AM, Ginn PE, Mansell JEKL, et al: Ulcerative facial and nasal dermatitis and stomatitis in cats associated with feline herpesvirus 1. *Vet Dermatol* 10: 267–274, 1999.

Hervás J, Chacon-Manrique de Lara F, Lopez J, et al: Granulomatous (pseudotumoral) iridociclitis associated with leishmaniasis in a cat. *Vet Rec* 149: 624–625, 2001.

Holland JL, Outerbridge CA, Affolter VK, et al: Detection of feline herpesvirus 1 DNA in skin biopsy specimens from cats with and without dermatitis. *J Am Vet Med Assoc* 229: 1442–1446, 2006.

Latimer Cl, Dunstan RW: Eosinophilic plaque involving eyelids of a cat. *J Am Anim Hosp Assoc* 23: 649–653, 1987.

Leiva M, Lloret A, Peña T, et al: Therapy of ocular and visceral leishmaniasis in a cat. *Vet Ophthalmol* 8: 71–75, 2005.

Lowenstein CL, Beck W, Bessman K, et al: Feline demodicosis caused by concurrent infestation with *Demodex cati* and an unnamed species of mite. *Vet Rec* 157: 290–292, 2005.

Martin CL, Stiles J, Willis M: Ocular adnexal cryptococcosis in a cat. *Vet Comp Ophthalmol* 6: 225–229, 1996.

McLaughlin SA: Iatrogenic blepharitis in a cat. *Fel Pract* 14: 39–41, 1982.

Moriello KA: Important factors in the pathogenesis of feline dermatophytosis. *Vet Med* 2003; 98: 845.

Moriello KA: Treatment of dermatophytosis in dogs and cats: Review of published studies. *Vet Dermatol* 15: 99–107, 2004.

Malik R, Hughes MS, Martin P, et al: Feline leprosy syndromes, in Greene CE (ed): Infectious Diseases of the Dog and Cat, 3rd ed. St Louis, WB Saunders, 2006, pp 477–480.

Takle GL, Hnilica KA: Eight emerging feline dermatoses. *Vet Med* 99: 456–465, 2004.

Cystadenoma

Cantaloube B, Raymond-Letron I, Regnier A: Multiple eyelid apocrine hidrocystomas in two Persian cats. *Vet Ophthalmol* 7: 121–125, 2004.

Chaitman J, van der Woerdt A, Bartick TE: Multiple eyelid cysts resembling apocrine hidrocystomas in three Persian cats and one Himalayan cat. *Vet Pathol* 36: 474–476, 1999.

Giudice C, Muscolo MC, Rondena M, et al: Eyelid multiple cysts of the apocrine gland of Moll in Persian cats. *J Feline Med Surg* 11: 487–491, 2009.

Sivagurunathan A, Goodhead AD, du Plessis EC: Multiple eyelid apocrine hidrocystoma in a domestic short-haired cat. *J S Afr Vet Assoc* 81: 65–68, 2010.

Yang SH, Liu CH, Hsu CD, et al: Use of chemical ablation with trichloroacetic acid to treat eyelid apocrine hidrocystomas in a cat. *J Am Vet Med Assoc* 230: 1170–1173, 2007.

Neoplasia

Abramo F, Pratesi F, Cantile C, et al: Survey of canine and feline follicular tumours and tumour-like lesions in central Italy. *J Small Anim Pract* 40: 479–481, 1999.

Aquino SM: Management of eyelid neoplasms in the dog and cat. *Clin Tech Small Anim Pract* 22: 46–54, 2007.

Bostock DE, Dye MT: Prognosis after surgical excision of fibrosarcomas in cats. *J Am Vet Med Assoc* 175: 727–728, 1979.

Buchholz J, Wergin M, Walt H, et al: Photodynamic therapy of feline cutaneous squamous cell carcinoma using a newly developed liposomal photosensitizer: Prelimary results concerning drug safety and efficacy. *J Vet Intern Med* 21: 770–775, 2007.

de Queiroz GF, Matera JM, Dagli MLZ: Clinical study of cryosurgery efficacy in the treatment of skin and subcutaneous tumors in dogs and cats. *Vet Surg* 37: 438–443, 2008.

Diters RW, Wlash KM: Feline basal cell tumors: a review of 124 cases. *Vet Pathol* 21: 51–56, 1984.

Doherty M: A bridge-flap blepharorrhaphy method of lower eyelid reconstruction in the cat. *J Am Anim Hosp Assoc* 9: 238–241, 1973.

Ghisleni G, Roccabianca P, Ceruti R, et al: Correlation between fine-needle aspiration cytology and histopathology in the evaluation of cutaneous and subcutaneous masses from dogs and cats. *Vet Clin Pathol* 35: 24–30, 2006.

Gomes LAM, Ferreira AMR, deAlmeida LEF, et al: Squamous cell carcinoma associated with actinic dermatitis in seven white cats. *Feline Pract* 28: 14–16, 2000.

Hagard GM: Eyelid reconstruction using a split eyelid flap after excision of a palpebral tumour in a Persian cat. *J Small Anim Pract* 46: 389–392, 2005.

Hardman C, Stanley R: Radioactive gold-198 seeds for the treatment of squamous cell carcinoma in the eyelid of a cat. *Aust Vet J* 79: 604–608, 2001.

Hartley C, Ladlow J, Smith KC: Cutaneous haemangiosarcoma of the lower eyelid in an elderly white cat. *J Feline Med Surg* 9: 78–81, 2007.

Hoffman A, Blocker T, Dubielzig R, et al: Feline periocular peripheral nerve sheath tumor: A case series. *Vet Ophthalmol* 8: 153–158, 2005.

Hunt GB: Use of the lip-to-lid flap for replacement of the lower eyelid in five cats. *Vet Surg* 35: 284–286, 2006.

McAbee KP, Ludwig LL, Bergman PJ, et al: Feline cutaneous hemangiosarcoma: a retrospective study of 18 cases (1998–2003). *J Am Anim Hosp Assoc* 41: 110–116, 2005.

McLaughlin SA, Whitley RD, Gilger BC, et al: Eyelid neoplasms in cats: A review of demographic data (1979–1989). *J Am Anim Hosp Assoc* 29: 63–67, 1993.

Montgomery KW, van der Woerdt A, Aquino SM, et al: Periocular cutaneous mast cell tumors in cats: Evaluation of surgical excision (33 cases). *Vet Ophthalmol* 13: 26–30, 2010.

Morgan RV: Procedures for excising eyelid masses and replacing a prolapsed third eyelid gland. *Vet Med* 99: 374–383, 2004.

Neumann SM: Palpebral squamous cell carcinoma in a cat. *Mod Vet Pract* 63: 547–548, 1982.

Newkirk KM, Rohrbach BW: A retrospective study of eyelid tumors from 43 cats. *Vet Pathol* 46: 916–927, 2009.

Riis RC, Vitali CM, Simons KB: Eyelid tumors, in Peiffer RL, Simons KB (eds): *Ocular tumors in animals and humans*. Ames, Iowa State Press, 2002, pp 25–86.

Schulman FY, Johnson TO, Facemire PR, et al: Feline peripheral nerve sheath tumors: Histologic, immunohistochemical, and clinicopathologic correlation (59 tumors in 53 cats). *Vet Pathol* 46: 1166–1180, 2009.

Spugnini EP, Vincenzi B, Citro G, et al: Electrochemotherapy for the treatment of squamous cell carcinoma in cats: a preliminary report. *Vet J* 179: 117–120, 2009.

Stell AJ, Dobson JM, Langmack K: Photodynamic therapy of feline superficial squamous cell carcinoma using topical 5-aminolaevulinic acid. *J Small Anim Pract* 42: 164–169, 2001.

Stockhaus C, Teske E, Rudolph R, et al: Assessment of cytological criteria for diagnosing basal cell tumors in the dog and cat. *J Small Anim Pract* 42: 582–586, 2001.

Turrell JM, Farrelly J, Page RL, et al: Evaluation of strontium 90 irradiation in treatment of cutaneous mast cell tumors in cats: 35 cases (1992–2002). *J Am Vet Med Assoc* 228: 898–901, 2006.

Wilcock BP, Yager JA, Zink MC: The morphology and behavior of feline cutaneous mastocytomas. *Vet Pathol* 23: 320–324, 1986.

Williams LW, Gelatt KN, Gwin RM: Ophthalmic neoplasms in the cat. *J Am Anim Hosp Assoc* 17: 999–1008, 1981.

CONJUNCTIVA

Dermoid

Barnett KC: Inherited eye disease in the dog and cat. *J Small Anim Pract* 29: 462–475, 1988.

Carter J, Himes R: Epibulbar dermoid involving the sclera, conjunctiva and eyelid in a cat. *J Am Anim Hosp Assoc* 7: 14–15, 1971.

Glaze MB: Congenital and hereditary ocular abnormalities in cats. *Clin Tech Small Anim Pract* 20: 74–82, 2005.

Hendy-Ibbs PM: Familial feline epibulbar dermoids. *Vet Rec* 116: 13–14, 1985.

Labue RH, Jones BR, Johnstone AC: Congenital dermoid in a cat. *N Z Vet J* 33: 154, 1985.

Rochat MC, Campbell GA, Panciera RJ: Dermoid cysts in cats: two cases and a review of the literature. *J Vet Diagn Invest* 8: 505–507, 1996.

Symblepharon

Andrew SE: Ocular manifestations of feline herpesvirus. *J Feline Med Surg* 3: 9–16, 2001.

Jacobi S, Dubielzig RR: Feline early life ocular disease. *Vet Ophthalmol* 11: 166–169, 2008.

Spiess B: Symblepharon, pseudopterygium and partial ankyloblepharon as consequences of feline herpesvirus keratoconjunctivitis. *Kleintierpraxis* 30: 149, 1985.

Infectious Conjunctivitis

Herpesvirus

Low HC, Powell CC, Veir JK, et al: Prevalence of feline herpesvirus 1, *Chlamydophila felis* and *Mycoplasma* spp DNA in conjunctival cells collected from cats with and without conjunctivitis. *Am J Vet Res* 68: 643–648, 2007.

Nasisse MP, Guy JS, Stevens JB, et al: Clinical and laboratory findings in chronic conjunctivitis in cats: 91 cases (1983-1991). *J Am Vet Med Assoc* 203: 834–837, 1993.

Stiles J, Townsend WM, Rogers QR, et al: Effect of oral administration of L-lysine on conjunctivitis caused by feline herpesvirus in cats. *Am J Vet Res* 63: 99–103, 2002.

Stiles J, McDermott M, Bigsby D, et al: Use of nested polymerase chain reaction to identify feline herpesvirus in ocular tissue from clinically normal cats and cats with corneal sequestra or conjunctivitis. *Am J Vet Res* 58: 338–342, 1997.

Stiles J, McDermott M, Willis M, et al: Comparison of nested polymerase chain reaction, virus isolation, and fluorescent antibody testing for identifying feline herpesvirus in cats with conjunctivitis. *Am J Vet Res* 58: 804–807, 1997.

Volopich S, Benetka V, Schwendenwein I, et al: Cytological findings and feline herpesvirus DNA and *Chlamydophila felis* antigen detection rates in normal cats and cats with conjunctival and corneal lesions. *Vet Ophthalmol* 8: 25–32, 2005.

Chlamydophila

Cello RM: Ocular infections in animals with PLT (Bedsonia) group agents. *Am J Ophthalmol* 63: 244–247, 1967.

Cello RM: Microbiological and immunologic aspects of feline pneumonitis. *J Am Vet Med Assoc* 158: 932–938, 1971.

Dean R, Harley R, Helps C, et al: Use of quantitative real-time PCR to monitor the response of *Chlamydophila felis* infection to doxycycline treatment. *J Clin Microbiol* 43: 1858–1864, 2005.

Gunn-Moore DA, Werrett G, Harbour DA, et al: Prevalence of *Chlamydia psittaci* antibodies in healthy pet cats in Britain. *Vet Rec* 136: 366–367, 1995.

Hoover EA, Kahn DE, Langloss JM: Experimentally induced feline chlamydial infection (feline pneumonitis). *Am J Vet Res* 39: 541–547, 1978.

Johnson FW: Isolation of *Chlamydia psittaci* from nasal and conjunctival exudates of a domestic cat. *Vet Rec* 114: 342–344, 1984.

McDonald M, Willett BJ, Jarrett O, et al: A comparison of DNA amplification, isolation and serology for detection of *Chlamydia psittaci* infection in cats. *Vet Rec* 143: 97–101, 1998.

O'Dair HA, Hopper CD, Gruffydd-Jones TJ, et al: Clinical aspects of *Chlamydia psittaci* infection in cats infected with feline immunodeficiency virus. *Vet Rec* 134: 365–368, 1994.

Owen WM, Sturgess CP, Harbour DA, et al: Efficacy of azithromycin for the treatment of feline chlamydophilosis. *J Feline Med Surg* 5: 305–311, 2003.

Rampazzo A, Appino S, Pregel P, et al: Prevalence of *Chlamydophila felis* and feline herpesvirus 1 in cats with conjunctivitis in northern Italy. *J Vet Intern Med* 17: 799–807, 2003.

Ramsey DT: Feline chlamydia and calicivirus infections. *Vet Clin North Amer Small Am Pract* 30: 1015–1028, 2000.

Shewen PE, Povey RC, Wilson MR: Feline chlamydial infection. *Can Vet J* 19: 289–292, 1978.

Sparkes AH, Caney SM, Sturgess CP, et al: The clinical efficacy of topical and systemic therapy for the treatment of feline ocular chlamydiosis. *J Feline Med Surg* 1: 31–35, 1999.

Studdert MJ, Studdert VP, Wirth HJ: Isolation of *Chlamydia psittaci* from cats with conjunctivitis. *Aust Vet J* 57: 515–517, 1981.

Sturgess CP, Gryffydd-Jones TJ, Harbour DA, et al: Controlled study of the efficacy of clavulanic acid-potentiated amoxicillin in the treatment of *Chlamydia psittaci* in cats. *Vet Rec* 149: 73–76, 2001.

Sykes JE: Feline chlamydiosis. *Clin Tech Small Anim Pract* 20: 129–134, 2005.

Sykes JE: Feline chlamydiosis, in Bonagura JD, Twedt DC (eds): *Kirk's Current Veterinary Therapy XIV.* St Louis, Saunders, 2009, pp 1185–1187.

Sykes JE: Feline upper respiratory tract pathogens: *Chlamydophila felis. Compend Contin Educ Vet* 23: 231–240, 2001.

Sykes JE, Anderson GA, Studdert VP, et al: Prevalence of feline *Chlamydia psittaci* and feline herpesvirus 1 in cats with upper respiratory tract disease. *J Vet Intern Med* 13: 153–162, 1999.

Sykes JE, Studdert VP, Browning GF: Polymerase chain reaction detection of *Chlamydia psittaci* in untreated and doxycycline-treated experimentally infected cats. *J Vet Intern Med* 13: 146–152, 1999.

TerWee J, Sabara M, Kokjohn K, et al: Characterization of the systemic disease and ocular signs induced by experimental infection with *Chlamydia psittaci* in cats. *Vet Microbiol* 59: 259–281, 1998.

Von Bomhard W, Polkinghorne A, Lu ZH, et al: Detection of novel chlamydiae in cats with ocular disease. *Am J Vet Res* 64: 1421–1428, 2003.

Wills J, Gruffydd-Jones TJ, Richmond S, et al: Isolation of *Chlamydia psittaci* from cases of conjunctivitis in a colony of cats. *Vet Rec* 114: 344–346, 1984.

Wills JM, Gruffydd-Jones TJ, Richmond SD, et al: Effect of vaccination on infection due to feline *Chlamydia psittaci. Infect Immun* 55: 2653–2657, 1987.

Mycoplasma

Blackmore DK, Hill A: The experimental transmission of various mycoplasmas of feline origin to domestic cats (*Felis catus*). *J Small Anim Pract* 14: 7–13, 1973.

Blackmore DK, Hill A, Jackson OF: The incidence of mycoplasma in pet and colony maintained cats. *J Small Anim Pract* 12: 207–217, 1971.

Campbell LH, Snyder SB, Reed C, et al: *Mycoplasma felis*-associated conjunctivitis in cats. *J Am Vet Med Assoc* 163: 991–995, 1973.

Cello RM: Association of pleuropneumonia-like organisms with conjunctivitis of cats. *Am J Ophthalmol* 43: 296–297, 1957.

Haesebrouck F, Devriese LA, van Rijssen B, et al: Incidence and significance of isolation of *Mycoplasma felis* from conjunctival swabs of cats. *Vet Microbiol* 26: 95–101, 1991.

Hartmann AD, Hawley J, Werckenthin C, et al: Detection of bacterial and viral organisms from the conjunctiva of cats with conjunctivitis and upper respiratory tract disease. *J Feline Med Surg* 12: 775–782, 2010.

Lavach JD, Thrall MA, Benjamin MM, et al: Cytology of normal and inflamed conjunctivas in dogs and cats. *J Am Vet Med Assoc* 170: 722–727, 1977.

Low HC, Powell CC, Veir JK, et al: Prevalence of feline herpesvirus 1, *Chlamydophila felis* and *Mycoplasma* spp DNA in conjunctival cells collected from cats with and without conjunctivitis. *Am J Vet Res* 68: 643–648, 2007.

Sandmeyer LS, Waldner CL, Bauer BS, et al: Comparison of polymerase chain reaction tests for diagnosis of feline herpesvirus, *Chlamydophila felis*, and *Mycoplasma* spp infection in cats with ocular disease in Canada. *Can Vet J* 51: 629–633, 2010.

Tan RJ, Miles JA: Characterization of mycoplasmas isolated from cats with conjunctivitis. *N Z Vet J* 21: 27–32, 1973.

Miscellaneous Agents

Campbell LH, Fox JG, Snyder SB: Ocular bacteria and mycoplasma of the clinically normal cat. *Feline Pract* 3: 10–12, 1973.

Espinola MB, Lilenbaum W: Prevalence of bacteria in the conjunctival sac and on the eyelid margin of clinically normal cats. *J Small Anim Pract* 37: 364–366, 1996.

Fox JG, Galus CB: Salmonella-associated conjunctivitis in a cat. *J Am Vet Med Assoc* 171: 845–847, 1977.

Gerding PA, Kakoma I: Microbiology of the canine and feline eye. *Vet Clin North Am Small Anim Pract* 20: 615–625, 1990.

Lamagna B, Paciello O, Ragozzino M, et al: Isolated lepromatous conjunctivo-corneal granuloma in a cat from Italy. *Vet Ophthalmol* 12: 97–101, 2009.

Omerod E, McCandlish IA, Jarrett O: Diseases produced by feline caliciviruses when administered to cats by aerosol or intranasal instillation. *Vet Rec* 104: 65–69, 1979.

Samuelson DA, Andresen TL, Gwin RM: Conjunctival fungal flora in horses, cattle, dogs, and cats. *J Am Vet Med Assoc* 184: 1240–1242, 1984.

Shewen PE, Povey RC, Wilson MR: A survey of the conjunctival flora of clinically normal cats and cats with conjunctivitis. *Can Vet J* 21: 231–233, 1980.

Allergic

Glaze MB: Ocular allergy. *Semin Vet Med Surg (Small Anim)* 6: 296–302, 1991.

Eosinophilic Conjunctivitis

Allgoewer I, Schaffer EH, Stockhaus C, et al: Feline eosinophilic conjunctivitis. *Vet Ophthalmol* 4: 69–74, 2001.

Hodges A: Eosinophilic keratitis and keratoconjunctivitis in a 7-year-old domestic shorthaired cat. *Can Vet J* 46: 1034–1035, 2005.

Larocca RD: Eosinophilic conjunctivitis, herpesvirus and mast cell tumor of the third eyelid in a cat. *Vet Ophthalmol* 3: 221–225, 2000.

Pentlarge VW: Eosinophilic conjunctivitis in five cats. *J Am Anim Hosp Assoc* 27: 21–28, 1991.

Lipogranulomatous Conjunctivitis

Kerline RL, Dubielzig RR: Lipogranulomatous conjunctivitis in cats. *Vet Comp Ophthalmol* 7: 177–179, 1997.

Read RA, Lucas J: Lipogranulomatous conjunctivitis: clinical findings from 21 eyes in 13 cats. *Vet Ophthalmol* 4: 93–98, 2001.

Thelaziasis

Knapp SE, Bailey RB, Bailey DE: Thelaziasis in cats and dogs—a case report. *J Am Vet Med Assoc* 138: 537–538, 1961.

Neoplasia

Cook CS, Rosenkrantz W, Peiffer RL, et al: Malignant melanoma of the conjunctiva in a cat. *J Am Vet Med Assoc* 186: 505–506, 1985.

Holt E, Goldschmidt MH, Skorupski K: Extranodal conjunctival Hodgkin's-like lymphoma in a cat. *Vet Ophthalmol* 9: 141–144, 2006.

Patnaik AK, Mooney S: Feline melanoma: A comparative study of ocular, oral and dermal neoplasms. *Vet Pathol* 25: 105–112, 1988.

Payen G, Estrada M, Clerc B, et al: A case of conjunctival melanoma in a cat. *Vet Ophthalmol* 11: 401–405, 2008.

Perlmann E, da Silva EG, Guedes PM, et al: Co-existing squamous cell carcinoma and hemangioma on the ocular surface of a cat. *Vet Ophthalmol* 13: 63–66, 2010.

Pirie CG, Dubielzig RR: Feline conjunctival hemangioma and hemangiosarcoma: A retrospective evaluation of eight cases (1993–2004). *Vet Ophthalmol* 9: 227–231, 2006.

Radi ZA, Miller DL, Hines ME: B-cell conjunctival lymphoma in a cat. *Vet Ophthalmol* 7: 413–415, 2004.

Schobert CS, Labelle P, Dubielzig RR: Feline conjunctival melanoma: histopathological characteristics and clinical outcomes. *Vet Ophthalmol* 13: 43–46, 2010.

Zaher AR, Miller DL, Hines ME: B-cell lymphoma in a cat. *Vet Ophthalmol* 7: 413–415, 2004.

Diagnostics

Lavach JD, Thrall MA, Benjamin MM, et al: Cytology of normal and inflamed conjunctivas in dogs and cats. *J Am Vet Med Assoc* 170: 722–727, 1977.

Willis M, Bounous D, Hirsh S, et al: Conjunctival brush cytology: evaluation of a new cytological collection technique in dogs and cats with a comparison to conjunctival scraping. *Vet Comp Ophthalmol* 7: 74–81, 1997.

LACRIMAL APPARATUS

Excretory

Anthony JMG, Sandmeyer LS, Laycock AR: Nasolacrimal obstruction caused by root abscess of the upper canine in a cat. *Vet Ophthalmol* 13: 106–109, 2010.

Covitz D, Hunziker J, Koch SA: Conjunctivorhinostomy: A surgical method for the control of epiphora in the dog and cat. *J Am Vet Med Assoc* 171: 251–255, 1977.

Gelatt KN, Cure TH, Guffy MM, et al: Dacryocystorhinography in the dog and cat. *J Small Anim Pract* 13: 381–397, 1972.

Secretory

Arnett BD, Brightman AH: Mussleman EE: Effect of atropine sulfate on tear production in the cat when used with ketamine hydrochloride and acetylpromazine maleate. *J Am Vet Med Assoc* 185: 214–215, 1984.

Brown MH, Brightman AH, Butine MD, et al: The phenol red thread tear test in healthy cats. *Vet Comp Ophthalmol* 7: 249–252, 1997.

Cullen CL, Lim C, Sykes J: Tear film breakup times in young healthy cats before and after anesthesia. *Vet Ophthalmol* 8: 159–165, 2005.

Cullen CL, Njaa BL, Grahn BH: Ulcerative keratitis associated with qualitative tear film abnormalities in cats. *Vet Ophthalmol* 2: 197–204, 1999.

Gwin RM, Gelatt KN, Peiffer RL: Parotid duct transposition in a cat with keratoconjunctivitis sicca. *J Am Anim Hosp Assoc* 13: 42–45, 1977.

Hacker DV: "Crocodile tears" syndrome in a domestic cat: Case report. *J Am Anim Hosp Assoc* 26: 245–246, 1990.

Johnson BW, Whiteley HE, McLaughlin SA: Effects of inflammation and aqueous tear film deficiency on conjunctival morphology and ocular mucus composition in cats. *Am J Vet Res* 51: 820–824, 1990.

Kern TJ, Erb HN: Facial neuropathy in dogs and cats: 95 cases (1975-1985). *J Am Vet Med Assoc* 191: 1604–1609.

McLaughlin SA, Brightman AH, Helper LC, et al: Effect of removal of the lacrimal and third eyelid glands on Schirmer tear tests in the cat. *J Am Vet Med Assoc* 193: 820–822, 1988.

Veith LA, Cure TH, Gelatt KN: The Schirmer tear test – in cats. *Mod Vet Pract* 51: 48–49, 1970.

NICTITATING MEMBRANE

Anatomy/Physiology

Nuyttens JJ, Simoens PJ: Morphologic study of the musculature of the third eyelid in the cat (*Felis catus*). *Lab Anim Sci* 45: 561–563, 1995.

Protrusion

Muir P, Harbour DA, Gruffydd-Jones TJ, et al: A clinical and microbiological study of cats with protruding nictitating membranes and diarrhea: Isolation of a novel virus. *Vet Rec* 127: 324–330, 1990.

Glandular Prolapse

Albert RA, Garrett PD, Whitley RD: Surgical correction of everted third eyelid in two cats. *J Am Vet Med Assoc* 180: 763–766, 1982.

Chahory S, Crasta M, Trio S, et al: Three cases of prolapse of the nictitans gland in cats. *Vet Ophthalmol* 7: 417–419, 2004.

Christmas R: Surgical correction of congenital ocular and nasal dermoids and third eyelid gland prolapse in related Burmese kittens. *Can Vet J* 33: 265–266, 1992.

Koch SA: Congenital ophthalmic abnormalities in the Burmese cat. *J Am Vet Med Assoc* 174: 90–91, 1979.

Schoofs SH: Prolapse of the gland of the third eyelid in a cat: A case report and literature review. *J Am Anim Hosp Assoc* 35: 240–242, 1999.

Horner's Syndrome

Baines SJ, Langley-Hobbs S: Horner's syndrome associated with a mandibular symphyseal fracture and bilateral temporomandibular luxation. *J Small Anim Pract* 42: 607–610, 2001.

Fox JG, Gutnick MJ: Horner's syndrome and brachial paralysis due to lymphosarcoma in a cat. *J Am Vet Med Assoc* 160: 977–980, 1972.

Frye FL: Horner's syndrome in a cat following cervical trauma. *Vet Med Small Anim Clin* 1973; 68: 754.

Holland CT: Horner's syndrome and ipsilateral laryngeal hemiplegia in three cats. *J Small Anim Pract* 37: 442–446, 1996.

Jones BR, Studdert VP: Horner's syndrome in the dog and cat as an aid to diagnosis. *Aust Vet J* 51: 329–332, 1975.

Kern TJ, Aromando MC, Erb HN: Horner's syndrome in cats and dogs: 100 cases (1975–1985). *J Am Vet Med Assoc* 195: 369–373, 1989.

Kneller SK, Lewis RE, Oliver JE: Horner's syndrome following common carotid artery catheterization in cats. *J Small Anim Pract* 13: 595–599, 1972.

Manning PD: Horner's syndrome secondary to metastatic squamous cell carcinoma of a retropharyngeal lymph node in a cat. *Aust Vet J* 76: 322–324, 1998.

Morgan RV, Zanotti SW: Horner's syndrome in dogs and cats: 49 cases (1980–1986). *J Am Vet Med Assoc* 194: 1096–1099, 1989.

Van den Broek AHM: Horner's syndrome in cats and dogs: A review. *J Small Anim Pract* 28: 929–940, 1987.

Eosinophilic

Keil SM, Olivero DK, McKeever PJ, et al: Bilateral nodular eosinophilic granulomatous inflammation of the nictitating membrane of a cat. *Vet Comp Ophthalmol* 7: 258–262, 1997.

Neoplasia

Buyukmihci N: Fibrosarcoma of the nictitating membrane in a cat. *J Am Vet Med Assoc* 167: 934–935, 1975.

Crafts GA, Pulley LT: Generalized cutaneous mast cell tumor in a cat. *Fel Pract* 5: 57–58, 1975.

Komaromy AM, Ramsey DT, Render JA, et al: Primary adencarcinoma of the gland of the nictitating membrane in a cat. *J Am Anim Hosp Assoc* 33: 333–336, 1997.

Larocca RD: Eosinophilic conjunctivitis, herpesvirus and mast cell tumor of the third eyelid in a cat. *Vet Ophthalmol* 3: 221–225, 2000.

Multari D, Vascellari M, Mutinelli F: Hemangiosarcoma of the third eyelid in a cat. *Vet Ophthalmol* 5: 273–276, 2002.

CORNEA

Reviews

Andrew SE: Immune-mediated canine and feline keratitis. *Vet Clin North Am Small Anim Pract* 38: 269–290, 2008.

Moore PA: Feline corneal disease. *Clin Tech Small Anim Pract* 20: 83–93, 2005.

Anatomy/Physiology

Blocker T, van der Woerdt A: A comparison of corneal sensitivity between brachycephalic and domestic short-haired cats. *Vet Ophthalmol* 4: 127–130, 2001.

Carrington SD, Woodward EG: Corneal thickness and diameter in the domestic cat. *Ophthal Physiol Optics* 3: 823–826, 1986.

Franzen AA, Pigatto JAT, Abib FC, et al: Use of specular microscopy to determine corneal endothelial cell morphology and morphometry in enucleated cat eyes. *Vet Ophthalmol* 13: 222–226, 2010.

Herring IP, Troy GC, Toth TE, et al: Feline leukemia virus detection in corneal tissues of cats by polymerase chain reaction and immunohistochemistry. *Vet Ophthalmol* 4: 119–126, 2001.

Kafarnik C, Fritsche J, Reese S: Corneal innervation in mesocephalic and brachycephalic dogs and cats: assessment using *in vivo* confocal microscopy. *Vet Ophthalmol* 11: 363–367, 2008.

Karfarnik C, Fritsche J, Reese S: *In vivo* confocal microscopy in the normal corneas of cats, dogs, and birds. *Vet Ophthalmol* 10: 222–230, 2007.

Moodie KL, Hashizume N, Houston DL, et al: Postnatal development of corneal curvature and thickness in the cat. *Vet Ophthalmol* 4: 267–272, 2001.

Schoster JV, Wickman L, Stuhr C: The use of ultrasonic pachymetry and computer enhancement to illustrate the collective corneal thickness profile of 25 cats. *Vet Comp Ophthalmol* 5: 68–73, 1995.

Corneal Opacities

Dystrophy

Carrington SD: Lipid keratopathy in a cat. *J Small Anim Pract* 24: 495–505, 1983.

Cooley PL, Dice PF: Corneal dystrophy in the dog and cat. *Vet Clin North Am Small Anim Pract* 20: 681–692, 1990.

Crispin S: Corneal dystrophies in small animals. *Vet Ann* 22: 298–310, 1982.

Godfrey VL, Nasisse MP: Corneal-endothelial dystrophy in a cat. *Trans Am Coll Vet Pathol* 242: 1985.

Jones BR: Inherited hyperchylomicronaemia in the cat. *J Small Anim Pract* 34: 493–499, 1993.

Kipnis RM: Keratopathy in a Siamese cat. *Fel Pract* 5: 33–36, 1975.

Olin DD, TenBroeck TJ: Corneal dystrophy in a cat. *Vet Med Small Anim Clin* 78: 1237–1238, 1973.

Florida spots

Peiffer R, Jackson W: Mycotic keratopathy of the dog and cat in the southeastern United States: A preliminary report. *J Am Anim Hosp Assoc* 15: 93–97, 1979.

Storage disease

Aguirre G, Stramm L, Haskins M: Feline mucopolysaccharidosis VI: General ocular and pigment epithelial pathology. *Invest Ophthalmol Vis Sci* 24: 991–1007, 1983.

Blakemore WF: A case of mannosidosis in the cat: clinical and histopathological findings. *J Small Anim Pract* 27: 447–455, 1986.

Blakemore WF: Neurolipidoses: examples of lysosomal storage diseases. *Vet Clin North Am Small Anim Pract* 10: 81–90, 1980.

Breton L, Guerin P, Morin M: A case of mycopolysaccharidosis VI in a cat. *J Am Anim Hosp Assoc* 19: 891–896, 1983.

Cork LC, Munnell JR, Lorenz MD: The pathology of feline GM2 gangliosidosis. *Am J Pathol* 90: 723–724, 1978.

Cowell K, Jezyk P, Haskins M, et al: Mucopolysaccharidosis in a cat. *J Am Vet Med Assoc* 169: 334–339, 1976.

Evans RJ: Lysosomal storage disease in dogs and cats. *J Small Anim Pract* 30: 144–150, 1989.

Haskins ME, Aguirre GD, Jezyk PF, et al: The pathology of the feline model of mucopolysaccharidosis VI. *Am J Pathol* 101: 657–674, 1980.

Haskins ME, Jezyk PF, Desnick RJ, et al: Mucopolysaccharidosis in a domestic shorthaired cat, a disease distinct from that seen in the Siamese cat. *J Am Vet Med Assoc* 175: 384–387, 1979.

Hubler M, Haskins ME, Arnold S, et al: Mucolipidosis type II in a domestic shorthair cat. *J Small Anim Pract* 37: 435–441, 1996.

Jezyk PF, Haskins ME, Newman LR: Alpha-mannosidosis in a Persian cat. *J Am Vet Med Assoc* 189: 1483–1485, 1986.

Jezyk PF, Haskins ME, Patterson DF, et al: Mucopolysaccharidosis in a cat with arylsulfatase B deficiency: A model of Maroteaux-Lamy syndrome. *Science* 198: 834–836, 1977.

Langweiler M, Haskins M, Jezyk P: Mucopolysaccharidosis in a litter of cats. *J Am Anim Hosp Assoc* 14: 748–751, 1978.

Murray JA, Blakemore WF, Barnett KC: Ocular lesions in cats with GM1-gangliosidosis with visceral involvement. *J Small Anim Pract* 18: 1–10, 1977.

Neuwelt EA, Johnson WG, Blank NK, et al: Characterization of a new model of GM2-gangliosidosis (Sandhoff's disease) in Korat cats. *J Clin Invest* 76: 482–490, 1985.

Stramm LE, Desnick RJ, Haskins ME, et al: Arylsulfatase B activity in cultured retinal pigment epithelium: Regional studies in feline mucopolysaccharidosis VI. *Invest Ophthalmol Vis Sci* 27: 1050–1057, 1986.

Wenger DA, Sattler M, Kudoh T, et al: Niemann-Pick disease: A genetic model in Siamese cats. *Science* 208: 1471–1473, 1980.

Yamato O, Matsunaga S, Takata K, et al: GM2-gangliosidosis variant O (Sandhoff-like disease) in a family of Japanese domestic cats. *Vet Rec* 155: 739–744, 2004.

Relapsing polychondritis

Bunge MM, Foil CS, Taylor HW, et al: Relapsing polychondritis in a cat. *J Am Anim Hosp Assoc* 28: 203–206, 1992.

Delmage DA, Kelly DF: Auricular chondritis in a cat. *J Small Anim Pract* 42: 499–501, 2001.

Gerber B, Crottaz M, von Tscharner C, et al: Feline relapsing polychondritis: Two cases and a review of the literature. *J Feline Med Surg* 4: 189–194, 2002.

Endothelial Dysfunction

Donaldson D, Billson FM, Scase TJ, et al: Congenital hyposomatotropism in a domestic shorthair cat presenting with congenital corneal oedema. *J Small Anim Pract* 49: 306–309, 2008.

Manx Dystrophy

Bistner SI, Aguirre G, Shively JN: Hereditary corneal dystrophy in the Manx cat: A preliminary report. *Invest Ophthalmol Vis Sci* 15: 15–26, 1976.

Infectious Keratitis

Herpesvirus

Beaumont SL, Maggs DJ, Clarke HE: Effects of bovine lactoferrin on *in vitro* replication of feline herpesvirus. *Vet Ophthalmol* 6: 245–250, 2003.

Bodle JE: Feline herpesvirus infection. *Surv Ophthalmol* 21: 209–215, 1976.

Burgesser KM, Hotaling S, Schiebel A, et al: Comparison of PCR, virus isolation, and indirect fluorescent antibody staining in the detection of naturally occurring feline herpesvirus infections. *J Vet Diagn Invest* 11: 122–126, 1999.

Drazenovich TL, Fascetti AJ, Westermeyer HD, et al: Effects of dietary lysine supplementation on upper respiratory and ocular disease and detection of infectious organisms in cats within an animal shelter. *Am J Vet Res* 70: 1391–1400, 2009.

Fontenelle JP, Powell CC, Veir JK, et al: Effect of topical ophthalmic application of cidofovir on experimentally induced primary ocular feline herpesvirus-1 infection in cats. *Am J Vet Res* 69: 289–293, 2008.

Galle LE: Antiviral therapy for ocular viral disease. *Vet Clin North Am Small Anim Pract* 34: 639–653, 2004.

Galle LE, Moore CP: Clinical microbiology, in Gelatt KN (ed): Veterinary Ophthalmology, 4th ed. Ames IA, Blackwell Publishing, 2007, pp 236–270.

Gaskell R, Dawson S, Radford A, et al: Feline herpesvirus. *Vet Res* 38: 337–354, 2007.

Gaskell RM, Povey RC: Experimental induction of feline viral rhinotracheitis virus re-excretion in FVR-recovered cats. *Vet Rec* 12: 128–133, 1977.

Gaskell RM, Povey RC: Feline viral rhinotracheitis: sites of virus replication and persistence in acutely and persistently infected cats. *Res Vet Sci* 27: 167–174, 1979.

Gaskell R, Dennis PE, Goddard LE, et al: Isolation of felid herpesvirus 1 from the trigeminal ganglia of latently infected cats. *J Gen Virol* 66: 391–394, 1985.

Haid C, Kaps S, Gonczi E, et al: Pretreatment with feline interferon omega and the course of subsequent infection with feline herpesvirus in cats. *Vet Ophthalmol* 10: 278–284, 2007.

Hara M, Fukuyama M, Suzuki Y, et al: Detection of feline herpesvirus 1 DNA by the nested polymerase chain reaction. *Vet Microbiol* 48: 345–352, 1996.

Hargis AM, Ginn PE, Mansell JEKL, et al: Ulcerative facial and nasal dermatitis and stomatitis in cats associated with feline herpesvirus 1. *Vet Dermatol* 10: 267–274, 1999.

Hartley C: Treatment of corneal ulcers. *What are the medical options? J Feline Med Surg* 12: 383–397, 2010.

Helps C, Reeves N, Egan K, et al: Detection of *Chlamydophila felis* and feline herpesvirus by multiplex real-time PCR analysis. *J Clin Microbiol* 41: 2734–2736, 2003.

Hussein ITM, Menashy RV, Field HJ: Penciclovir is a potent inhibitor of feline herpesvirus-1 with susceptibility determined at the level of virus-encoded thymidine kinase. *Antiviral Res* 78: 268–274, 2008.

Lappin MR, Veir JK, Satyaraj E, et al: Pilot study to evaluate the effect of oral supplementation of *Enterococcus faecium* SF68 on cats with latent feline herpesvirus 1. *J Feline Med Surg* 11: 650–654, 2009.

Lim CC, Reilly CM, Thomasy SM, et al: Effects of feline herpesvirus type 1 on tear film break-up time, Schirmer tear test results, and conjunctival goblet cell density in experimentally infected cats. *Am J Vet Res* 70: 394–403, 2009.

Maggs DJ: Antiviral therapy for feline herpesvirus infections. *Vet Clin North Am Small Anim Pract* 40: 1055–1062, 2010.

Maggs DJ: Update on pathogenesis, diagnosis and treatment of feline herpesvirus type 1. *Clin Tech Small Anim Pract* 20: 94–101, 2005.

Maggs DJ, Clarke HE: Relative sensitivity of polymerase chain reaction assays used for detection of feline herpesvirus type 1 DNA in clinical samples and commercial vaccines. *Am J Vet Res* 66: 1550–1555, 2005.

Maggs DJ, Clark HE: *In vitro* efficacy of ganciclovir, cidofovir, penciclovir, foscarnet, idoxuridine, and acyclovir against feline herpesvirus-1. *Am J Vet Res* 65: 399–403, 2004.

Maggs DJ, Collins BK, Thorne JG, et al: Effects of L-lysine and L-arginine on *in vitro* replication of feline herpesvirus type-1. *Am J Vet Res* 61: 1474–1478, 2000.

Maggs DJ, Lappin MR, Nasisse MP: Detection of feline herpesvirus-specific antibodies and DNA in aqueous humor from cats with or without uveitis. *Am J Vet Res* 60: 932–936, 1999.

Maggs DJ, Lappin MR, Reif JS, et al: Evaluation of serologic and viral detection methods for diagnosing feline herpesvirus-1 infection in cats with acute respiratory tract or chronic ocular disease. *J Am Vet Med Assoc* 214: 502–507, 1999.

Maggs DJ, Nasisse MP, Kass PH: Efficacy of oral supplementation with L-lysine in cats latently infected with feline herpesvirus. *Am J Vet Res* 64: 37–42, 2003.

Maggs DJ, Sykes JE, Clarke HE, et al: Effects of dietary lysine supplementation in cats with enzootic upper respiratory disease. *J Feline Med Surg* 9: 97–108, 2007.

Malik R, Lessels NS, Webb S, et al: Treatment of feline herpesvirus-1 associated disease in cats with famciclovir and related drugs. *J Feline Med Surg* 11: 40–48, 2009.

Nasisse MP: Feline herpesvirus ocular disease. *Vet Clin North Am Small Anim Pract* 20: 667–680, 1990.

Nasisse MP, Dorman DC, Jamison KC, et al: Effects of valacyclovir in cats infected with feline herpesvirus 1. *Am J Vet Res* 58: 1141–1144, 1997.

Nasisse MP, English RV, Tompkins MB, et al: Immunologic, histologic, and virologic features of herpesvirus-induced stromal keratitis in cats. *Am J Vet Res* 56: 51–55, 1995.

Nasisse MP, Glover TL, Moore CP, et al: Detection of feline herpesvirus 1 DNA in corneas of cats with eosinophilic keratitis or corneal sequestration. *Am J Vet Res* 59: 856–858, 1998.

Nasisse MP, Guy JS, Davidson MG, et al: Experimental ocular herpesvirus infection in the cat. Sites of virus replication, clinical features and effects of corticosteroid administration. *Invest Ophthalmol Vis Sci* 30: 1758–1768, 1989.

Nasisse MP, Guy JS, Davidson MG, et al: *In vitro* susceptibility of feline herpesvirus-1 to vidarabine, idoxuridine, trifluridine, acyclovir, or bromovinyldeoxyuridine. *Am J Vet Res* 50: 158–160, 1989.

Ohmura Y, Ono E, Matsuura, et al: Detection of feline herpesvirus 1 transcripts in trigeminal ganglia of latently infected cats. *Arch Virol* 129: 341–347, 1993.

Sandmeyer LS, Keller CB, Bienzle D: Effects of cidofovir on cell death and replication of feline herpesvirus-1 in cultured feline corneal epithelial cells. *Am J Vet Res* 66: 217–222, 2005.

Sandmeyer LS, Keller CB, Bienzle D: Effects of interferon-alpha on cytopathic changes and titers for feline herpesvirus-1 in primary cultures of feline corneal epithelial cells. *Am J Vet Res* 66: 210–216, 2005.

Siebeck N, Hurley DJ, Garcia M, et al: Effects of human recombinant alpha-2b interferon and feline recombinant omega interferon on in vitro replication of feline herpesvirus-1. *Am J Vet Res* 67: 1406–1411, 2006.

Sjödahl-Essén T, Tidholm A, Thorén P, et al: Evaluation of different sampling methods and results of real-time PCR for detection of feline herpes virus-1, *Chlamydophila felis* and *Mycoplasma felis* in cats. *Vet Ophthalmol* 11: 375–380, 2008.

Stiles J: Feline herpesvirus. *Vet Clin North Am Small Anim Pract* 30: 1001–1014, 2000.

Stiles J: Treatment of cats with ocular disease attributable to herpesvirus infection: 17 cases (1983-1993). *J Am Vet Med Assoc* 5: 599–603, 1995.

Stiles J, Pogranichniy R: Detection of virulent feline herpesvirus-1 in the corneas of clinically normal cats. *J Feline Med Surg* 10: 154–159, 2008.

Stiles J, Townsend WM: Feline ophthalmology, in Gelatt KN (ed): Veterinary Ophthalmology, 4th ed. Ames IA, Blackwell Publishing, 2007, pp 1095–1164.

Thiry E, Addie D, Belak S, et al: Feline herpesvirus infection. ABCD guidelines on prevention and management. *J Feline Med Surg* 11: 547–555, 2009.

Thomasy SM, Lim CC, Reilly CM, et al: Evaluation of orally administered famciclovir in cats experimentally infected with feline herpesvirus type-1. *Am J Vet Res* 2011; 72: 85-95.

Thomasy SM, Maggs DJ, Moulin NK, et al: Pharmacokinetics and safety of penciclovir following oral administration of famciclovir to cats. *Am J Vet Res* 68: 1252–1258, 2007.

Townsend WM, Stiles J, Guptill-Yoran L, et al: Development of a reverse transcriptase-polymerase chain reaction assay to detect feline herpesvirus-1 latency-associated transcripts in the trigeminal ganglia and corneas of cats that did not have clinical signs of ocular disease. *Am J Vet Res* 65: 314–319, 2004.

Verneuil M: Topical application of feline interferon omega in the treatment of herpetic keratitis in the cat: preliminary study. *Vet Ophthalmol* 2004; 7: 427.

Weigler B, Babineau C, Sherry B, et al: High sensitivity polymerase chain reaction assay for active and latent feline herpesvirus-1 infections in domestic cats. *Vet Rec* 140: 335–338, 1997.

Weigler BJ, Guy JS, Nasisse MP, et al: Effect of a live attenuated intranasal vaccine on latency and shedding of feline herpesvirus 1 in domestic cats. *Arch Virol* 142: 2389–2400, 1997.

Williams DL, Fitzmaurice T, Lay L, et al: Efficacy of antiviral agents in feline herpetic keratitis: Results of an *in vitro* study. *Curr Eye Res* 29: 215–218, 2004.

Williams DL, Robinson JC, Lay E, et al: Efficacy of topical acyclovir for the treatment of feline herpetic keratitis: Results of a prospective clinical trial and data from *in vitro* investigations. *Vet Rec* 157: 254–257, 2005.

Chlamydia/Mycoplasma

Gray LD, Ketring KL, Tang YW: Clinical use of 16S rRNA gene sequencing to identify *Mycoplasma felis* and *M.gateae* associated ulcerative keratitis. *J Clin Microbiol* 43: 3431–3434, 2005.

Von Bomhard W, Polkinghorne A, Lu ZH, et al: Detection of novel chlamydiae in cats with ocular disease. *Am J Vet Res* 64: 1421–1428, 2003.

Volopich S, Benetka V, Schwendenwein I, et al: Cytologic findings and feline herpesvirus DNA and *Chlamydophila felis* antigen detection rates in normal cats and cats with conjunctival and corneal lesions. *Vet Ophthalmol* 8: 25–32, 2005.

Fungal keratitis

Bernays ME, Peiffer RL: Ocular infections with dematiaceous fungi in two cats and a dog. *J Am Vet Med Assoc* 213: 507–509, 1998.

Labelle AL, Hamor RD, Barger AM, et al: *Aspergillus flavus* keratomycosis in a cat treated with topical 1% voriconazole solution. *Vet Ophthalmol* 12; 48–52, 2009.

Miller DM, Blue JL, Winston SM: Keratomycosis caused by *Cladosporium sp* in a cat. *J Am Vet Med Assoc* 182: 1121–1122, 1983.

Peiffer RL, Jackson WF: Mycotic keratopathy of the dog and cat in the southeastern United States: A preliminary report. *J Am Anim Hosp Assoc* 15: 93–97, 1979.

Miscellaneous agents

Buyukmihci N, Bellhorn RW, Hunziker J, et al: Encephalitozoon (Nosema) infection of the cornea in a cat. *J Am Vet Med Assoc* 171: 355–357, 1977.

Campbell LH, McCree AV: Corneal abscess in a cat: Treatment by subconjunctival antibiotics. *Feline Pract* 8: 30–31, 1978.

Lin C-T, Petersen-Jones SM: Antibiotic susceptibility of bacteria isolated from cats with ulcerative keratitis in Taiwan. *J Small Anim Pract* 49: 80–83, 2008.

Moore DL, Jones RG: Corneal stromal abscess in a cat. *J Small Anim Pract* 35: 432–434, 1994.

Richter M, Matheis F, Gonczi E, et al: *Parachlamydia acanthamoebae* in domestic cats with and without corneal disease. *Vet Ophthalmol* 13: 235–237, 2010.

Ulcerative Keratitis

Hartley C: Treatment of corneal ulcers: When is surgery indicated? *J Feline Med Surg* 12: 398–405, 2010.

Hartley C: Aetiology of corneal ulcers. Assume FHV-1 unless proven otherwise. *J Feline Med Surg* 12: 24–35, 2010.

LaCroix NC, van der Woerdt A, Olivero DK: Nonhealing corneal ulcers in cats: 29 cases (1991-1999). *J Am Vet Med Assoc* 218: 733–735, 2001.

Ledbetter EC, Scarlett JM: Isolation of obligate anaerobic bacteria from ulcerative keratitis in domestic animals. *Vet Ophthalmol* 2008: 11; 114–122.

Schmidt GM, Blanchard GL, Keller WF: The use of hydrophilic contact lenses in corneal diseases of the dog and cat: A preliminary report. *J Small Anim Pract* 18: 773–777, 1977.

Bullous Keratopathy

Glover TL, Nasisse MP, Davidson MG: Acute bullous keratopathy in the cat. *Vet Comp Ophthalmol* 4: 66–70, 1994.

Keratoconjunctivitis Sicca

Canapp SO, Cohn LA, Maggs DJ, et al: Xerostomia, xerophthalmia, and plasmacytic infiltrates of the salivary gland (Sjögren's-like syndrome) in a cat. *J Am Vet Med Assoc* 218: 59–65, 2001.

Lim CC, Cullen CL: Schirmer tear test values and tear film break-up times in cats with conjunctivitis. *Vet Ophthalmol* 8: 305–310, 2005.

Ghaffari MS, Malmasi A, Bokaie S: Effect of acepromazine or xylazine on tear production as measured by Schirmer tear test in normal cats. *Vet Ophthalmol* 13: 1–3, 2010.

Margadant DL, Kirkby K, Andrew SE, et al: Effect of topical tropicamide on tear production as measured by Schirmer's tear test in normal dogs and cats. *Vet Ophthalmol* 6: 315–320, 2003.

Eosinophilic Keratitis

Allgoewer I, Schaffer EH, Stockhaus C, et al: Feline eosinophilic conjunctivitis. *Vet Ophthalmol* 4: 69–74, 2001.

Andrew SE: Immune-mediated canine and feline keratitis. *Vet Clin North Am Small Anim Pract* 38: 269–290, 2008.

Bedford P: What is your diagnosis? Eosinophilic keratoconjunctivitis. *J Small Anim Pract* 1997; 38: 233, 270.

Bedford PGC, Cotchin E: An unusual chronic keratoconjunctivitis in the cat. *J Small Anim Pract* 24: 85–102, 1983.

Brightman AH, Vestre WA, Helper LC, et al: Chronic eosinophilic keratitis in the cat. *Feline Pract* 9: 21–23, 1979.

Chisholm WH: Feline eosinophilic keratitis. *Can Vet J* 1989; 30: 438.

Colitz CMH, Davidson MG, Gilger BC: Bilateral proliferative keratitis in a domestic long-haired cat. *Vet Ophthalmol* 5: 137–140, 2002.

Hodges A: Eosinophilic keratitis and keratoconjunctivitis in a 7-year-old domestic shorthaired cat. *Can Vet J* 46: 1034–1035, 2005.

Morgan RV, Abrams KL, Kern TJ: Feline eosinophilic keratitis: a retrospective study of 54 cases (1989–1994). *Vet Comp Ophthalmol* 6: 131–134, 1996.

Murphy JM: Exfoliative cytologic examination as an aid in diagnosing ocular diseases in the dog and cat. *Semin Vet Med Surg* 3: 10–14, 1988.

Nasisse MP, Glover TL, Moore CP, et al: Detection of feline herpesvirus I DNA in corneas of cats with eosinophilic keratitis or corneal sequestration. *Am J Vet Res* 59: 856–858, 1998.

Paulsen ME, Lavach JD, Severin GA, et al: Feline eosinophilic keratitis: A review of 15 cases. *J Am Anim Hosp Assoc* 23: 63–69, 1987.

Prasse KW, Winston SM: Cytology and histopathology of feline eosinophilic keratitis. *Vet Comp Ophthalmol* 6: 74–81, 1996.

Spiess AK, Sapienza JS, Mayordomo A: Treatment of proliferative eosinophilic keratitis with topical 1.5% cyclosporine: 35 cases. *Vet Ophthalmol* 12: 132–137, 2009.

Spiess BM, Leber A, von Beust BR, et al: Chronic eosinophilic keratitis in the cat. *Schweiz Arch Tierheilkd* 133: 113–118, 1991.

Sequestrum

Andrew SE, Tou S, Brooks DE: Corneoconjunctival transposition for the treatment of feline corneal sequestra: A retrospective study of 17 cases (1990–1998). *Vet Ophthalmol* 4: 107–111, 2001.

Barachetti L, Giudice C, Mortellaro CM: Amniotic membrane transplantation for the treatment of feline corneal sequestrum: Pilot study. *Vet Ophthalmol* 13: 326–330, 2010.

Blogg JR, Stanley RG, Dutton AG: Use of conjunctival pedicle grafts in the management of feline keratitis nigrum. *J Small Anim Pract* 30: 678–684, 1989.

Cullen CL, Wadowska DW, Singh A, et al: Ultrastructural findings in feline corneal sequestra. *Vet Ophthalmol* 8: 295–303, 2005.

Dalla F, Pisoni L, Masetti L: Feline corneal sequestration: a review of medical treatment in 37 cases. *Vet Res Commun* 31 (Suppl 1): 285–288, 2007.

Davidson HJ, Gerlach JA, Bull RW: Determination of protein concentrations and their molecular weight in tears from cats with normal corneas and cats with corneal sequestrum. *Am J Vet Res* 53: 1756–1759, 1992.

Ejima H, Hara N, Kajigaya H: Detection of iron in a blackish lesion in a case of feline corneal sequestration. *J Vet Med Sci* 55: 1051–1052, 1993.

Featherstone HJ, Franklin VJ, Sansom J: Feline corneal sequestrum: laboratory analysis of ocular samples from 12 cats. *Vet Ophthalmol* 7: 229–238, 2004.

Featherstone HJ, Sansom J: Feline corneal sequestra: A review of 64 cases (80 eyes) from 1993–2000. *Vet Ophthalmol* 7: 213–227, 2004.

Featherstone HJ, Sansom J, Heinrich CL: The use of porcine small intestinal submucosa in ten cases of feline corneal disease. *Vet Ophthalmol* 4: 147–153, 2001.

Gelatt KN: Corneal sequestration in a cat. *Vet Med Small Anim Clin* 66: 561–562, 1971.

Gelatt KN, Peiffer RL, Stevens J: Chronic ulcerative keratitis and sequestrum in the domestic cat. *J Am Anim Hosp Assoc* 9: 204–213, 1973.

Gemensky AJ, Wilkie DA: Mineralized corneal sequestrum in a cat. *J Am Vet Med Assoc* 219: 1568–1572, 2001.

Gimenez-Peña MTP, Farina IM: Lamellar keratoplasty for the treatment of feline corneal sequestrum. *Vet Ophthalmol* 1: 163–166, 1998.

Gionfriddo JR: An enlarging pigmented corneal mass in a cat. *Vet Med* 96: 438–443, 2001.

Grahn BH, Sisler S, Storey E: Qualitative tear film and conjunctival goblet cell assessment of cats with corneal sequestra. *Vet Ophthalmol* 8: 167–170, 2005.

Knecht CD, Schiller AG, Small E: Focal degeneration of the cornea with sequestration in a cat. *J Am Vet Med Assoc* 149: 1192–1193, 1966.

Morgan RV: Feline corneal sequestration: a retrospective study of 42 cases (1987–1991). *J Am Anim Hosp Assoc* 30: 24–30, 1994.

Pentlarge VW: Corneal sequestration in cats. *Compend Contin Educ Vet* 11: 24–32, 1989.

Souri E: The feline corneal nigrum. *Vet Med Small Anim Clin* 70: 531–534, 1975.

Startup FG: Corneal necrosis and sequestration in the cat: a review and record of 100 cases. *J Small Anim Pract* 29: 476–486, 1988.

Stiles J, McDermott M, Bigsby D, et al: Use of nested polymerase chain reaction to identify feline herpesvirus in ocular tissue from clinically normal cats and cats with corneal sequestra or conjunctivitis. *Am J Vet Res* 58: 338–342, 1997.

Townsend WM, Rankin AJ, Stiles J, et al: Heterologous penetrating keratoplasty for treatment of a corneal sequestrum in a cat. *Vet Ophthalmol* 11: 273–278, 2008.

Wagner F, Meyer-Lindendberg A, Heider HJ, et al: A comparison of corneal sensitivity between healthy cats and cats with corneal sequestra. *Berl Munch Tierarztl Wochenschr* 116: 427–431, 2003.

Volopich S, Benetka V, Schwendenwein I, et al: Cytologic findings, and feline herpesvirus DNA and *Chlamydophila felis* antigen detection rates in normal cats and cats with conjunctival and corneal lesions. *Vet Ophthalmol* 8: 25–32, 2005.

Staphyloma

Rampazzo A, Eule C, Speier S, et al: Scleral rupture in dogs, cats, and horses. *Vet Ophthalmol* 9: 149–155, 2006.

Skorobohach BJ, Hendrix DVH: Staphyloma in a cat. *Vet Ophthalmol* 6: 93–97, 2003.

Limbal Melanoma

Betton A, Healy LN, English RV, et al: Atypical limbal melanoma in a cat. *J Vet Intern Med* 13: 379–381, 1999.

Harling DE, Peiffer RL, Cook CS: Feline limbal melanoma: Four cases. *J Am Anim Hosp Assoc* 22: 795–802, 1986.

Kanai K, Kanemaki N, Matsuo S, et al: Excision of a feline limbal melanoma and use of nictitans cartilage to repair the resulting corneoscleral defect. *Vet Ophthalmol* 9: 255–258, 2006.

Plummer CE, Kallberg ME, Ollivier FJ, et al: Use of a biosynthetic material to repair the surgical defect following excision of an epibulbar melanoma in a cat. *Vet Ophthalmol* 11: 250–254, 2008.

Sullivan TC, Nasisse MP, Davidson MG, et al: Photocoagulation of limbal melanoma in dogs and cats: 15 cases (1989–1993). *J Am Vet Med Assoc* 208: 891–894, 1996.

Miscellaneous Masses

Smith J, Bistner S, Riis R: Infiltrative corneal lesions resembling fibrous histiocytoma: Clinical and pathological findings in six dogs and one cat. *J Am Vet Med Assoc* 169: 722–726, 1976.

Surgical Methods

Barros PSM, Safatle AMV, Godoy CA, et al: Amniotic membrane transplantation for the reconstruction of the ocular surface in three cases. *Vet Ophthalmol* 8: 189–192, 2005.

Bussieres M, Krohne SG, Stiles J, et al: The use of porcine small intestinal submucosa for the repair of full-thickness corneal defects in dogs, cats, and horses. *Vet Ophthalmol* 7: 352–359, 2004.

Featherstone HJ, Sansom J, Heinrich CL: The use of porcine small intestinal submucosa in ten cases of feline corneal disease. *Vet Ophthalmol* 4: 147–153, 2001.

Hansen PA, Guandalini A: A retrospective study of 30 cases of frozen lamellar corneal graft in dogs and cats. *Vet Ophthalmol* 2: 233–241, 1999.

Vanore M, Chahory S, Payen G, et al: Surgical repair of deep melting ulcers with porcine small intestinal submucosa (SIS) graft in dogs and cats. *Vet Ophthalmol* 10: 93–99, 2007.

Watté CM, Elks R, Moore DL, et al: Clinical experience with butyl-2-cyanoacrylate adhesive in the management of canine and feline corneal disease. *Vet Ophthalmol* 7: 319–326, 2004.

Anterior Uvea

Anatomy/Physiology

Bergsma DR, Brown KS: White fur, blue eyes, and deafness in the domestic cat. *J Hered* 62: 171–185, 1971.

Coulter DB, Martin CL, Alvarado TP: A cat with white fur and one blue eye. *Calif Vet* 9: 11–14, 1980.

Gelatt K, Boggess T, Cure T: Evaluation of mydriatics in the cat. *J Am Anim Hosp Assoc* 9: 283–287, 1973.

Schmidt KS, Hacker DV, Kass PH, et al: Effects of systemic administration of 0.5% tropicamide on intraocular pressure, pupillary diameter, blood pressure, and heart rate in normal cats. *Vet Ophthalmol* 9: 137–139, 2006.

Stadtbäumer K, Frommlet F, Nell B: Effects of mydriatics on intraocular pressure and pupil size in the normal feline eye. *Vet Ophthalmol* 9: 233–237, 2006.

Stadtbäumer K, Köstlin RG, Zahn KJ: Effects of topical 0.5% tropicamide on intraocular pressure in normal cats. *Vet Ophthalmol* 5: 107–112, 2002.

Thibos LN, Levick WR, Morstyn R: Ocular pigmentation in white and Siamese cats. *Invest Ophthal Vis Sci* 19: 475–486, 1980.

Dyscoria

Boydell P: Iatrogenic pupillary dilation resembling Pourfour du Petit syndrome in three cats. *J Small Anim Pract* 41: 202–203, 2000.

Collins BK, O'Brien D: Autonomic dysfunction of the eye. *Semin Vet Med Surg (Small Anim)* 5: 24–36, 1990.

Neer TM, Carter JD: Anisocoria in dogs and cats. *Compend Cont Educ Vet* 9: 817–823, 1987.

Nell B, Suchy A: 'D-shaped' and 'reverse-D-shaped' pupil in a cat with lymphosarcoma. *Vet Ophthalmol* 1: 53–56, 1998.

Dysautonomia

Barnett KC: Observations on the feline dilated pupil syndrome. *Vet Rec* 1984; 114: 351.

Bromberg NM, Cabaniss LD: Feline dysautonomia: A case report. *J Am Anim Hosp Assoc* 24: 106–108, 1988.

Cave TA, Knottenbelt C, Mellor DJ, et al: Outbreak of dysautonomia (Key-Gaskell syndrome) in a closed colony of pet cats. *Vet Rec* 153: 387–392, 2003.

Key TJ, Gaskell CJ: Puzzling syndrome in cats associated with pupillary dilation. *Vet Rec* 1982; 110: 160.

Nash AS, Griffiths IR, Sharp NJ: The Key-Gaskell syndrome – an autonomic polyganglionopathy. *Vet Rec* 111: 307–308, 1982.

Nunn F, Cave TA, Knottenbelt C, et al: Association between Key-Gaskell syndrome and infection by *Clostridium botulinum* type C/D. *Vet Rec* 155: 111–115, 2004.

Rochlitz I: Feline dysautonomia (the Key-Gaskell or dilated pupil syndrome): A preliminary report. *J Small Anim Pract* 25: 587–598, 1984.

Sharp NJH, Nash AS, Griffiths IR: Feline dysautonomia (the Key-Gaskell syndrome): A clinical and pathological study of 40 cases. *J Small Anim Pract* 25: 599–615, 1984.

Symonds HW, McWilliams P, Thompson H, et al: A cluster of cases of feline dysautonomia (Key-Gaskell syndrome) in a closed colony of cats. *Vet Rec* 136: 353–355, 1995.

Uveal Cysts

Belkin PV: Iris cysts in cats. *Feline Pract* 13: 12–18, 1983.

Peiffer RL: Iris cyst in a cat. *Feline Pract* 7: 15–17, 1977.

Gemensky-Metzler AJ, Wilkie DA, Cook CS: The use of semiconductor diode laser for deflation and coagulation of anterior uveal cysts in dogs, cats and horses: A report of 20 cases. *Vet Ophthalmol* 7: 360–368, 2004.

Anterior Uveitis

Reviews

Chavkin MJ, Lappin MR, Powell CC, et al: Seroepidemiologic and clinical observations of 93 cases of uveitis in cats. *Prog Vet Comp Ophthalmol* 2: 29–36, 1992.

Colitz CMH: Feline uveitis: Diagnosis and treatment. *Clin Tech Small Anim Pract* 20: 117–120, 2005.

Crispin SM: Uveitis associated with systemic disease in cats. *Feline Pract* 17: 16–24, 1987.

Crispin SM: Uveitis in the dog and cat. *J Small Anim Pract* 29: 429–447, 1988.

Cullen CL, Webb AA: Ocular manifestations of systemic diseases. Part 2: The cat, in Gelatt KN (ed): *Veterinary Ophthalmology*, 4th ed. Oxford, Blackwell, 2007, pp 1538–1587.

Davidson MG, Nasisse MP, English RV, et al: Feline anterior uveitis: A study of 53 cases. *J Am Anim Hosp Assoc* 27: 77–83, 1991.

Goodhead AD: Uveitis in dogs and cats: Guidelines for the practitioner. *J S Afr Vet Assoc* 67: 12–19, 1996.

Hakanson N, Forrester SD: Uveitis in the dog and cat. *Vet Clin North Am Small Anim Pract* 20: 715–735, 1990.

Lappin MR: Feline infectious uveitis. *J Feline Med Surg* 2: 159–163, 2000.

Lappin MR, Marks A, Greene CE, et al: Serologic prevalence of selected infectious disease in cats with uveitis. *J Am Vet Med Assoc* 201: 1005–1009, 1992.

Olin D: Examination of the aqueous humor as a diagnostic aid in anterior uveitis. *J Am Vet Med Assoc* 171: 557–559, 1977.

Peiffer RL, Wilcock BP: Histopathologic study of uveitis in cats: 139 cases (1978-1988). *J Am Vet Med Assoc* 198: 135–138, 1991.

Peiffer RL, Wilcock BP, Yin H: The pathogenesis and significance of pre-iridal fibrovascular membrane in domestic animals. *Vet Pathol* 27: 41–45, 1990.346.

Powell CC, Lappin MR: Causes of feline uveitis. *Compend Contin Educ Pract Vet* 23: 128–141, 2001.

Powell CC, Lappin MR: Diagnosis and treatment of feline uveitis. *Compend Contin Educ Pract Vet* 23: 258–266, 2001.

Rankin AJ, Krohne SG, Glickman NW, et al: Laser flaremetric evaluation of experimentally induced blood-aqueous barrier disruption in cats. *Am J Vet Res* 63: 750–756, 2002.

Stiles J: Ocular infections, in Greene CE (ed): *Infectious Diseases of the Dog and Cat*, 3rd ed. St Louis, Saunders, 2006, pp 974–991.

Stiles J, Townsend WM: Feline ophthalmology, in Gelatt KN (ed): *Veterinary Ophthalmology*, 4th ed. Ames IA, Blackwell Publishing, 2007, pp 1117–1124.

Townsend WM: Canine and feline uveitis. *Vet Clin North Am Small Anim Pract* 38: 323–346, 2008.

Feline leukemia virus

Albert DM: The role of viruses in the development of ocular tumors. *Ophthalmology* 87: 1219–1225, 1980.

Brightman AH, Macy DW, Gosselin Y: Pupillary abnormalities associated with the feline leukemia complex. *Feline Pract* 7: 23–27, 1977.

Brightman AH, Ogilvie GK, Tompkins M: Ocular disease in FeLV-positive cats: 11 cases (1981–1986). *J Am Vet Med Assoc* 198: 1049–1051, 1991.

Callanan JJ, McCandlish IA, O'Neil B, et al: Lymphosarcoma in experimentally induced feline immunodeficiency virus infection. *Vet Rec* 130: 293–295, 1992.

Willis AM: Feline leukemia virus and feline immunodeficiency virus. *Vet Clin North Am Small Anim Pract* 30: 971–986, 2000.

Feline imunodeficiency virus (FIV)

Davidson MG, Rottman JB, English RV, et al: Feline immunodeficiency virus predisposes cats to acute generalized toxoplasmosis. *Am J Pathol* 143: 1486–1497, 1993.

English RV, Davidson MG, Nasisse MP, et al: Intraocular disease associated with feline immunodeficiency virus infection in cats. *J Am Vet Med Assoc* 196: 1116–1119, 1990.

Loesenbeck G, Drommer W, Egberink HF, et al: Immunohistochemical findings in eyes of cats serologically positive for feline immunodeficiency virus (FIV). *Zentralbl Veterinarmed [B]*. 43: 305–311, 1996.

Loesenbeck G, Drommer W, Heider HJ: Findings in the eyes of serologically FIV (feline immunodeficiency virus) positive cats. *Dtsch Tierarztl Wochenschr* 102: 348–351, 1995.

O'Neill SA, Lappin MR, Reif JS, et al: Clinical and epidemiologic aspects of feline immunodeficiency virus and *Toxoplasma gondii* coinfections in cat. *J Am Anim Hosp Assoc* 198: 135–138, 1991.

Phillips TR, Prospero-Garcia O, Puaoi DL, et al: Neurological abnormalities associated with feline immunodeficiency virus infection. *J Gen Virol* 75: 979–987, 1994.

Witt CJ, Moench TR, Gittelsohn AM et al: Epidemiologic observations on feline immunodeficiency virus and *Toxoplasma gondii* coinfection in cats in Baltimore MD. *J Am Vet Med Assoc* 194: 229–233, 1989.

Feline infectious peritonitis (FIP)

Addie DD, Jarrett O: Feline coronavirus infections, in Greene CE (ed): *Infectious Diseases of the Dog and Cat*, 3rd ed. St Louis, Saunders, 2006, pp 88–102.

Andrew SE: Feline infectious peritonitis. *Vet Clin North Am Small Anim Pract* 30: 987–1000, 2000.

Campbell LH, Reed C: Ocular signs associated with feline infectious peritonitis in two cats. *Feline Pract* 5: 32–35, 1975.

Carlton WW, Lavignette AM, Szczech GM: A case of feline infectious peritonitis with ocular lesions. *J Am Anim Hosp Assoc* 9: 256–261, 1973.

Doherty MJ: Ocular manifestations of feline infectious peritonitis. *J Am Vet Med Assoc* 159: 417–424, 1971.

Foley JE, Lapointe JM, Koblik P, et al: Diagnostic features of clinical neurologic feline infectious peritonitis. *J Vet Intern Med* 12: 415–423, 1998.

Gelatt KN: Iridocyclitis-panophthalmitis associated with feline infectious peritonitis. *Vet Med Small Anim Clin* 68: 56–57, 1973.

Giori L, Giordano A, Guidice C, et al: Performances of different diagnostic tests for feline infectious peritonitis in challenging clinical cases. *J Small Anim Pract* 52: 152–157, 2011.

Hartmann K: Feline infectious peritonitis. *Vet Clin North Am Small Anim Pract* 35: 39–79, 2005.

Hartmann K, Binder C, Hirschberger J, et al: Comparison of different tests to diagnose feline infectious peritonitis. *J Vet Intern Med* 17: 781–790, 2003.

Hartmann K, Ritz S: Treatment of cats with feline infectious peritonitis. *Vet Immunol Immunopathol* 123: 172–175, 2008.

Hok K: Demonstration of feline infectious peritonitis virus in conjunctival epithelial cells from cats. *APMIS* 97: 820–824, 1989.

Ishida T, Shibanai A, Tanaka S, et al: Use of recombinant feline interferon and glucocorticoid in the treatment of feline infectious peritonitis. *J Feline Med Surg* 6: 107–109, 2004.

Kline KL, Joseph RJ, Averill DR: Feline infectious peritonitis with neurologic involvement: Clinical and pathological findings in 24 cats. *J Am Anim Hosp Assoc* 30: 111–118, 1994.

Kornegay JN: Feline infectious peritonitis: The central nervous system form. *J Am Anim Hosp Assoc* 14: 580–584, 1978.

Krehbiel JD, Sanger VL, Ravi A: Ophthalmic lesions in feline infectious peritonitis: Gross, microscopic and ultrastructural changes. *Vet Pathol* 11: 443–444, 1974.

McReynolds C, Macy D: Feline infectious peritonitis. Part I. Etiology and diagnosis. *Compend Contin Educ Vet* 19: 1007–1016, 1997.

Norris JM, Bosward KL, White JD, et al: Clinicopathological findings associated with feline infectious peritonitis in Sydney, Australia: 42 cases (1990–2002). *Aust Vet J* 83: 666–673, 2005.

Pedersen NC: A review of feline infectious peritonitis: 1963–2008. *J Feline Med Surg* 11: 225–258, 2009.

Rohrbach BW, Legendre AM, Baldwin CA, et al: Epidemiology of feline infectious peritonitis among cats examined at veterinary medical teaching hospitals. *J Am Vet Med Assoc* 218: 1111–1115, 2001.

Slauson OD, Finn JP: Meningoencephalitis and panophthalmitis in feline infectious peritonitis. *J Am Vet Med Assoc* 160: 729–734, 1972.

Weiss R: Treatment of feline infectious peritonitis with immunomodulating agents and antiviral drugs: A review. *Feline Pract* 23: 103–106, 1995.

Zenger E: FIP, FeLV, FIV: Making a diagnosis. *Feline Pract* 28: 16–18, 2000.

Toxoplasmosis

Bussanich MN, Rootman J: Implicating toxoplasmosis as the cause of ocular lesions. *Vet Med* 80: 43–46, 1985.

Burney DP, Chavkin MA, Dow SW, et al: Polymerase chain reaction for the detection of *Toxoplasma gondii* within aqueous humor of experimentally-inoculated cats. *Vet Parasitol* 79: 181–186, 1998.

Campbell LH, Schiessl MM: Ocular manifestations of toxoplasmosis, infectious peritonitis, and lymphosarcoma in cats. *Mod Vet Pract* 59: 761–764, 1978.

Chavkin MJ, Lappin RM, Powell CC, et al: *Toxoplasma gondii*-specific antibodies in the aqueous humor of cats with toxoplasmosis. *Am J Vet Res* 55: 1244–1249, 1994.

Davidson MG: Toxoplasmosis. *Vet Clin North Am Small Anim Pract* 30: 1051–1062, 2000.

Davidson MG, English RV: Feline ocular toxoplasmosis. *Vet Ophthalmol* 1: 71–80, 1998.

Davidson MG, English RV, Rottman J, et al: Feline immunodeficiency virus predisposes cats to secondary acute generalized toxoplasmosis: A model for AIDS. *Am J Pathol* 143: 1486–1497, 1993.

Davidson MG, Lappin MR, English RV, et al: A feline model of ocular toxoplasmosis. *Invest Ophthalmol Vis Sci* 34: 3653–3660, 1993.

Davidson MG, Lappin MR, Rottman JR, et al: Paradoxical effect of clindamycin in experimental, acute toxoplasmosis in cats. *Antimicrob Agents Chemother* 40: 1352–1359, 1996.

Dubey JP: Persistence of *Toxoplasma gondii* in the tissues of chronically infected cats. *J Parasitol* 63: 156–157, 1977.

Dubey JP, Carpenter JL: Histologically confirmed clinical toxoplasmosis in cats: 100 cases (1952-1990). *J Am Vet Med Assoc* 203: 1556–1566, 1993.

Dubey JP, Johnstone I: Fatal neonatal toxoplasmosis in cats. *J Am Anim Hosp Assoc* 18: 461–467, 1982.

Engstrom RE, Holland RB, Nussenblatt RB, et al: Current practices in the management of ocular toxoplasmosis. *Am J Ophthalmol* 111: 601–610, 1991.

Hill SL, Lappin MR, Carman J, et al: Comparison of methods for estimation of *Toxoplasma gondii*-specific antibody production in the aqueous humor of cats. *Am J Vet Res* 56: 1181–1186, 1995.

Hirth RS, Nielsen SW: Pathology of feline toxoplasmosis. *J Small Anim Pract* 10: 213–221, 1969.

Lappin MR, Burney DP, Dow SW, et al: Polymerase chain reaction for the detection of *Toxoplasma gondii* in aqueous humor of cats. *Am J Vet Res* 57: 1589–1593, 1996.

Lappin MR, Burney DP, Hill SA, et al: Detection of *Toxoplasma gondii*-specific IgA in the aqueous humor of cats. *Am J Vet Res* 1995; 56: 774–778.

Lappin MR, Chavkin MJ, Munana KR, et al: Feline ocular and cerebrospinal fluid *Toxoplasma gondii*-specific humoral immune responses following specific and nonspecific immune stimulation. *Vet Immunol Immunopathol* 55: 23–31, 1996.

Lappin MR, Greene CE, Prestwood AK, et al: Diagnosis of recent *Toxoplasma gondii* infection in cats by use of an enzyme-linked immunosorbent assay for immunoglobulin M. *Am J Vet Res* 50: 1580–1586, 1989.

Lappin MR, Greene CE, Winston S, et al: Clinical feline toxoplasmosis. Serologic diagnosis and therapeutic management of 15 cases. *J Vet Intern Med* 3: 139–143, 1989.

Lappin MR, Roberts SM, Davidson MG, et al: Enzyme-linked immunosorbent assays for the detection of *Toxoplasma gondii*-specific antibodies and antigens in the aqueous humor of cats. *J Am Vet Med Assoc* 201: 1010–1016, 1992.

Pearce J, Giuliano EA, Galle LE, et al: Management of bilateral uveitis in a *Toxoplasma gondii*-seropositive cats with histopathologic evidence of fungal panuveitis. *Vet Ophthalmol* 10: 216–221, 2007.

Piper RC, Cole CR, Shadduck JA: Natural and experimental ocular toxoplasmosis in animals. *Am J Ophthalmol* 69: 662–668, 1970.

Powell CC, Lappin MR: Clinical ocular toxoplasmosis in neonatal kittens. *Vet Ophthalmol* 4: 87–92, 2001.

Stile J, Prade R, Greene C: Detection of *Toxoplasma gondii* in feline and canine biological samples by use of polymerase chain reaction. *Am J Vet Res* 57: 264–267, 1996.

Vainisi SJ, Campbell LH: Ocular toxoplasmosis in cats. *J Am Vet Med Assoc* 154: 141–152, 1969.

Systemic Mycoses

Reviews

Davies C, Troy GC: Deep mycotic infections in cats. *J Am Anim Hosp Assoc* 32: 380–391, 1996.

Foy DS, Trepanier LA: Antifungal treatment of small animal veterinary patients. *Vet Clin North Am Small Anim Pract* 40: 1171–1188, 2010.

Gionfriddo JR: Feline systemic fungal infections. *Vet Clin North Am Small Anim Pract* 30: 1029–1050, 2000.

Histoplasmosis

Aronson E, Bendickson JC, Miles KG, et al: Disseminated histoplasmosis with osseous lesions in a cat with feline lymphosarcoma. *Vet Radiol* 27: 50–53, 1986.

Breitschwerdt EB, Halliwell WH, Burk RL, et al: Feline histoplasmosis. *J Am Anim Hosp Assoc* 13: 216–222, 1977.

Clinkenbeard KD, Cowell RL, Tyler RD: Disseminated histoplasmosis in cats: 12 cases (1981–1986). *J Am Vet Med Assoc* 190: 1445–1448, 1987.

Gwin RM, Makley TA, Wyman M, et al: Multifocal ocular histoplasmosis in a dog and cat. *J Am Vet Med Assoc* 176: 638–642, 1980.

Hodges RD, Legendre AM, Adams LG, et al: Itraconazole for the treatment of histoplasmosis in cats. *J Vet Intern Med* 8: 409–413, 1994.

Johnson LR, Fry MM, Anez KL, et al: Histoplasmosis infection in two cats from California. *J Am Anim Hosp Assoc* 40: 165–169, 2004.

Noxon JO, Digilro K, Schmidt DA: Disseminated histoplasmosis in a cat: Successful treatment with ketaconazole. *J Am Vet Med Assoc* 181: 817–820, 1982.

Pearce J, Giuliano EA, Galle LE, et al: Management of bilateral uveitis in a *Toxoplasma gondii*-seropositive cat with histopathologic evidence of fungal panuveitis. *Vet Ophthalmol* 10: 216–221, 2007.

Peiffer RL: Ocular manifestations of disseminated histoplasmosis in a cat. *Feline Pract* 9: 24–29, 1979.

Percy DH: Feline histoplasmosis with ocular involvement. *Vet Pathol* 18: 163–169, 1981.

Wolf AM, Belden NM: Feline histoplasmosis. A literature review and retrospective study of 20 new cases. *J Am Anim Hosp Assoc* 20: 995–998, 1984.

Cryptococcosis

Blouin P, Cello RM: Experimental ocular cryptococcosis: Preliminary studies in cats and mice. *Invest Ophthalmol Vis Sci* 19: 21–30, 1980.

Dye JA, Campbell KL: Cutaneous and ocular cryptococcosis in a cat: Case report and literature review. *Comp Anim Pract* 2: 34–42, 1988.

Fischer CA: Intraocular cryptococcosis in two cats. *J Am Vet Med Assoc* 158: 191–198, 1971.

Flatland B, Greene RT, Lappin MR: Clinical and serologic evaluation of cats with cryptococcosis. *J Am Vet Med Assoc* 209: 1110–1113, 1996.

Gerds-Grogan S, Dayrell-Hart B: Feline cryptococcosis: a retrospective evaluation. *J Am Anim Hosp Assoc* 33: 118–122, 1997.

Gwin RM, Gelatt KN, Hardy R, et al: Ocular cryptococcosis in a cat. *J Am Anim Hosp Assoc* 13: 680–684, 1977.

Jacobs GJ, Medleau L, Calvert C, et al: Cryptococcal infection in cats: Factors influencing treatment outcome, and results of sequential serum antigen titers in 35 cats. *J Vet Intern Med* 11: 1–4, 1997.

Malik R, Vogelnest L, O'Brien CR, et al: Infections and some other conditions affecting the skin and subcutis of the naso-ocular region of cats – clinical experience 1987–2003. *J Feline Med Surg* 6: 383–390, 2004.

Pentlarge VW, Martin RA: Treatment of cryptococcosis in three cats, using ketoconazole. *J Am Vet Med Assoc* 188: 536–538, 1986.

Rosenthal JJ, Heidgerd J, Peiffer RL: Ocular and systemic cryptococcosis in a cat. *J Am Anim Hosp Assoc* 17: 307–310, 1981.

Schulman J: Ketoconazole for successful treatment of cryptococcosis in a cat. *J Am Vet Med Assoc* 187: 508–509, 1985.

Wilkinson GT: Feline cryptococcosis: A review and seven case reports. *J Small Anim Pract* 20: 749–768, 1979.

Blastomycosis

Alden CL, Mohan R: Ocular blastomycosis in a cat. *J Am Vet Med Assoc* 164: 527–528, 1974.

Breider MA, Walker TL, Legendre AM, et al: Blastomycosis in cats: Five cases (1979–1986). *J Am Vet Med Assoc* 193: 570–572, 1988.

Gilor C, Graves TK, Barger AM, et al: Clinical aspects of natural infection with *Blastomyces dermatitidis* in cats: 8 cases (1991-2005). *J Am Vet Med Assoc* 229: 96–99, 2006.

Miller PE, Miller LM, Schoster JV: Feline blastomycosis: A report of three cases and literature review (1961–1988). *J Am Anim Hosp Assoc* 26: 417–424, 1990.

Nasisse MP, van Ee RT, Wright B: Ocular changes in a cat with disseminated blastomycosis. *J Am Vet Med Assoc* 187: 629–631, 1985.

Coccidioidomycosis

Angell JA, Shively JN, Merideth RE, et al: Ocular coccidioidomycosis in a cat. *J Am Vet Med Assoc* 187: 167–169, 1985.

Graupmann-Kuzma A, Valentine BA, Shubitz LF, et al: Coccidioidomycosis in dogs and cats: A review. *J Am Anim Hosp Assoc* 44: 226–235, 2008.

Greene RT, Troy GC: Coccidioidomycosis in 48 cats: A retrospective study (1984–1993). *J Vet Intern Med* 9: 86–91, 1995.

Reed RE, Hoge RS, Trautman RJ: Coccidioidomycosis in two cats. *J Am Vet Med Assoc* 143: 953–956, 1963.

Tofflemire K, Betbeze C: Three cases of feline ocular coccidioidomycosis: presentation, clinical features, diagnosis, and treatment. *Vet Ophthalmol* 13: 166–172, 2010.

Miscellaneous mycoses

Gerding PA, Morton LD, Dye JA: Ocular and disseminated candidiasis in an immunosuppressed cat. *J Am Vet Med Assoc* 204: 1635–1638, 1994.

Miller WW, Albert RA: Ocular and systemic candidiasis in a cat. *J Am Anim Hosp Assoc* 24: 521–524, 1988.

Bartonellosis

Fontanelle J, Powell CC, Hill A, et al: Prevalence of serum antibodies against Bartonella species in the serum of cats with or without uveitis. *J Feline Med Surg* 10: 41–46, 2008.

Guptill L: Feline bartonellosis. *Vet Clin North Am Small Anim Pract* 40: 1073–1090, 2010.

Ketring KL, Zuckerman EE, Hardy WD: Bartonella: A new etiological agent of feline ocular disease. *J Am Anim Hosp Assoc* 40: 6–12, 2004.

Kordick DL, Papich MG, Breitschwerdt EB: Efficacy of enrofloxacin or doxycycline for treatment of *Bartonella henselae* or *Bartonella clarridgeiae* infection in cats. *Antimicrob Agents Chemother* 41: 2448–2455, 1997.

Lappin MR, Black JC: *Bartonella spp* infection as a possible cause of uveitis in a cat. *J Am Vet Med Assoc* 214: 1205–1207, 1999.

Lappin MR, Kordick DL, Breitschwerdt EB: *Bartonella spp* antibodies and DNA in aqueous humour of cats. *J Feline Med Surg* 2: 61–68, 2000.

Powell CC, McInnis CL, Fontenelle JP, et al: *Bartonella* species, feline herpesvirus-1, and *Toxoplasma gondii* PCR assay results from blood and aqueous humor samples from 104 cats with naturally occurring endogenous uveitis. *J Feline Med Surg* 12: 923–928, 2010.

Parasitic

Bussanich MN, Rootman J: Intraocular nematode in a cat. *Feline Pract* 13: 24–26, 1983.

Harris BP, Miller PE, Bloss JR, et al: Ophthalmomyiasis interna anterior associated with *Cuterebra spp* in a cat. *J Am Vet Med Assoc* 216: 352–355, 2000.

Johnson BW, Helper LC, Szajerski ME: Intraocular Cuterebra in a cat. *J Am Vet Med Assoc* 193: 829–830, 1988.

Stiles J, Rankin A: Ophthalmomyiasis interna anterior in a cat: Surgical resolution. *Vet Ophthalmol* 9: 165–168, 2006.

Other agents

Breitschwerdt EB, Abrams-Ogg AC, Lappin MR, et al: Molecular evidence supporting *Ehrlichia canis*-like infection in cats. *J Vet Intern Med* 16: 642–649, 2002.

Dietrich U, Arnold P, Guscetti F, et al: Ocular manifestation of disseminated *Mycobacterium simiae* infection in a cat. *J Small Anim Pract* 44: 121–125, 2003.

Lubin JR, Albert DM, Essex M, et al: Experimental anterior uveitis after subcutaneous injection of feline sarcoma virus. *Invest Ophthalmol Vis Sci* 24: 1055–1062, 1983.

Trauma

Brightman AH, Szajerski ME: Traumatic endophthalmitis in the cat. *Feline Pract* 14: 7–9, 1984.

Vestre WA, Brightman AH: Traumatic hyphema in a cat. *Feline Pract* 10: 36–37, 1980.

Lens-Induced

Davidson MG, Nasisse MP, Jamieson VE, et al: Traumatic anterior lens capsule disruption. *J Am Anim Hosp Assoc* 27: 410–414, 1991.

Dubielzig RR, Ketring KL, McLellan GJ, Albert DM: Septic implantation syndrome, in Veterinary Ocular Pathology. St Louis, Saunders, 2010, pp 94, 98–99, 335, 337.

Neoplasia

Reviews

Acland G: Intraocular tumors in dogs and cats. *Compend Cont Educ Vet* 1: 558–566, 1979.

Grahn BH, Peiffer RL, Cullen CL, et al: Classification of feline intraocular neoplasms based on morphology, histochemical staining, and immuno-histochemical labeling. *Vet Ophthalmol* 9: 395–403, 2006.

Dubielzig RR: Ocular neoplasia in small animals. *Vet Clin North Am Small Anim Pract* 20: 837–848, 1990.

Williams LW, Gelatt KN, Gwin RM: Ophthalmic neoplasms in the cat. *J Am Anim Hosp Assoc* 17: 999–1008, 1981.

Diffuse iris melanoma

Acland GM, McLean IW, Aguirre GD, et al: Diffuse iris melanoma in cats. *J Am Vet Med Assoc* 176: 52–56, 1980.

Albert DM, Shadduck JA, Craft JL, et al: Feline uveal melanoma model induced with feline sarcoma virus. *Invest Ophthalmol Vis Sci* 20: 606–624, 1981.

Bellhorn RW, Henkind P: Intraocular malignant melanoma in domestic cats. *J Small Anim Pract* 10: 631–637, 1969.

Bertoy RW, Brightman AL, Regan K: Intraocular melanoma with multiple metastases in a cat. *J Am Vet Med Assoc* 192: 87–89, 1988.

Bjerkas E, Arnesen K, Peiffer RL: Diffuse amelanotic iris melanoma in a cat. *Vet Comp Ophthalmol* 7: 190–191, 1997.

Cardy RH: Primary intraocular malignant melanoma in a Siamese cat. *Vet Pathol* 14: 648–649, 1977.

Cullen CL, Haines DM, Jackson ML, et al: Lack of detection of feline leukemia and feline sarcoma viruses in diffuse iris melanomas of cats by immunohistochemistry and polymerase chain reaction. *J Vet Diag Invest* 14: 340–343, 2002.

Day MJ, Lucke VM: Melanocytic neoplasia in the cat. *J Small Anim Pract* 36: 207–213, 1995.

Duncan DE, Peiffer RL: Morphology and prognostic indicators of anterior uveal melanomas in cats. *Prog Vet Comp Ophthalmol* 1: 25–32, 1991.

Harris BP, Dubielzig RR: Atypical primary ocular melanoma in cats. *Vet Ophthalmol* 2: 121–124, 1999.

Kalishman JB, Chappell R, Flood LA, et al: Matched observational study of survival in cats with enucleation due to diffuse iris melanoma. *Vet Ophthalmol* 1: 25–29, 1998.

Patnaik AK, Mooney S: Feline melanoma: a comparative study of ocular, oral and dermal neoplasms. *Vet Pathol* 25: 105–112, 1988.

Peiffer RL, Seymour WG, Williams LW: Malignant melanoma of the iris and ciliary body in a cat. *Mod Vet Pract* 58: 854–856, 1977.

Planellas M, Pastor J, Torres M, et al: Unusual presentation of a metastatic uveal melanoma in a cat. *Vet Ophthalmol* 13: 391–394, 2010.

Stiles J, Bienzle D, Render JA, et al: Use of nested polymerase chain reaction (PCR) for detection of retroviruses from formalin-fixed, paraffin-embedded uveal melanomas in cats. *Vet Ophthalmol* 2: 113–116, 1999.

Miscellaneous neoplasms

Dubielzig RR, Steinberg H, Garvin H, et al: Iridociliary epithelial tumors in 100 dogs and 17 cats: A morphological study. *Vet Ophthalmol* 1: 223–231, 1998.

Evans PM, Lynch GL, Dubielzig RR: Anterior uveal spindle cell tumor in a cat. *Vet Ophthalmol* 13: 387–390, 2010.

Labelle P, Holmberg BJ: Ocular myxoid leiomyosarcoma in a cat. *Vet Ophthalmol* 13: 58–62, 2010.

Michau TM, Proulx DR, Rushton SD, et al: Intraocular extramedullary plasmacytoma in a cat. *Vet Ophthalmol* 6: 177–181, 2003.

Miller WW, Boosinger TR: Intraocular osteosarcoma in a cat. *J Am Anim Hosp Assoc* 23: 317–320, 1987.

Peiffer RL: Ciliary body epithelial tumors in the dog and cat: A report of thirteen cases. *J Small Anim Pract* 24: 347–370, 1983.

Peiffer RL, Monticello T, Bouldin TW: Primary ocular sarcomas in the cat. *J Small Anim Pract* 29: 105–116, 1988.

Lymphoma

Campbell DH, Schiessl MM: Ocular manifestations of toxoplasmosis, infectious peritonitis, and lymphosarcoma in cats. *Mod Vet Pract* 59: 761–764, 1978.

Carlton WW: Intraocular lymphosarcoma. Two cases in Siamese cats. *J Am Anim Hosp Assoc* 12: 83–87, 1976.

Corcoran KA, Peiffer RL, Koch SA: Histopathologic features of feline ocular lymphosarcoma: 49 cases (1978–1992). *Vet Comp Ophthalmol* 5: 35–41, 1995.

Couto GC: What is new on feline lymphoma? *J Feline Med Surg* 3: 171–176, 2001.

Meincke JE: Reticuloendothelial malignancies, with intraocular involvement in the cat. *J Am Vet Med Assoc* 148: 157–161, 1966.

Slatter DH, Taylor RF, Brobst DF: Ocular manifestations of myeloproliferative disease in a cat. *Aust Vet J* 50: 164–168, 1974.

Taylor SS, Goodfellow MR, Browne WJ, et al: Feline extranodal lymphoma: Response to chemotherapy and survival in 110 cats. *J Small Anim Pract* 50: 584–592, 2009.

Metastatic neoplasia

Bellhorn RW: Secondary ocular adenocarcinoma in three dogs and a cat. *J Am Vet Med Assoc* 160: 302–307, 1972.

Cassotis NJ, Dubielzig RR, Gilger BC, et al: Angioinvasive pulmonary carcinoma with posterior segment metastasis in four cats. *Vet Ophthalmol* 2: 125–131, 1999.

Cook CS, Peiffer RL, Stine PE: Metastatic ocular squamous cell carcinoma in a cat. *J Am Vet Med Assoc* 185: 1547–1549, 1984.

Dubielzig RR, Grendahl RL, Orcutt JC, et al: Metastases, in Peiffer RL, Simons KB (eds): *Ocular Tumors in Animals and Humans*. Ames, Iowa State Press, 2002, pp 337–378.

Gionfriddo JR, Fix AS, Niyo Y, et al: Ocular manifestations of a metastatic pulmonary adenocarcinoma in a cat. *J Am Vet Med Assoc* 197: 372–374, 1990.

Hamilton HB, Severin GA, Nold J: Pulmonary squamous cell carcinoma with intraocular metastasis in a cat. *J Am Vet Med Assoc* 185: 307–309, 1984.

Hayden DW: Squamous cell carcinoma in a cat with intraocular and orbital metastases. *Vet Pathol* 13: 332–336, 1976.

Moise NS, Riis RC, Allison NM: Ocular manifestations of metastatic sweat gland adenocarcinoma in a cat. *J Am Vet Med Assoc* 180: 1100–1103, 1982.

Murphy CJ, Canton DC, Bellhorn RW, et al: Disseminated adenocarcinoma with ocular involvement in a cat. *J Am Vet Med Assoc* 195: 488–491, 1989.

O'Rourke MD, Geib LW: Endometrial adenocarcinoma in a cat. *Cornell Vet* 60: 598–604, 1970.

West CS, Wolf ED, Vainisi SJ: Intraocular metastasis of mammary adenocarcinoma in the cat. *J Am Anim Hosp Assoc* 15: 725–728, 1979.

Post-traumatic sarcoma

Barrett PM, Merideth RE, Alarcon FL: Central amaurosis induced by an intraocular, posttraumatic fibrosarcoma in a cat. *J Am Anim Hosp Assoc* 31: 242–245, 1995.

Carter RT, Giudice C, Dubielzig RR, et al: Telomerase activity with concurrent loss of cell cycle regulation in feline post-traumatic ocular sarcomas. *J Comp Pathol* 133: 235–245, 2005.

Cullen CL, Haines DM, Jackson ML, et al: The use of immunohistochemistry and the polymerase chain reaction for detection of feline leukemia virus and feline sarcoma virus in six cases of feline ocular sarcoma. *Vet Ophthalmol* 1: 189–193, 1998.

Dubielzig RR: Ocular sarcoma following trauma in three cats. *J Am Vet Med Assoc* 184: 578–581, 1984.

Dubielzig RR, Everitt J, Shadduck JA, et al: Clinical and morphologic features of post-traumatic ocular sarcomas in cats. *Vet Pathol* 27: 62–65, 1990.

Dubielzig RR, Hawkins KL, Toy KA, et al: Morphologic features of feline ocular sarcomas in 10 cats: light microscopy, ultrastructure, and immunohistochemistry. *Vet Comp Ophthalmol* 4: 7–12, 1994.

Hakanson N, Shively JN, Reed RE, et al: Intraocular spindle cell sarcoma following ocular trauma in a cat: case report and literature review. *J Am Anim Hosp Assoc* 26: 63–66, 1990.

Woog J, Albert DM, Gonder JR, et al: Osteosarcoma in a phthisical feline eye. *Vet Pathol* 20: 209–214, 1983.

Zeiss CJ, Johnson EM, Dubielzig RR: Feline intraocular tumors may arise from transformation of lens epithelium. *Vet Pathol* 40: 355–362, 2003.

Therapeutic Reviews

Giuliano E: Nonsteroidal anti-inflammatory drugs in veterinary ophthalmology. *Vet Clin North Am Small Anim Pract* 34: 707–723, 2004.

Holmberg B, Maggs D: The use of corticosteroids to treat ocular inflammation. *Vet Clin North Am Small Anim Pract* 34: 693–705, 2004.

Wilkie DA: Control of ocular inflammation. *Vet Clin North Am Small Anim Pract* 20: 693–713, 1990.

GLAUCOMA

Anatomy/Physiology

Aubin ML, Powell CC, Gionfriddo JR, et al: Ultrasound biomicroscopy of the feline anterior segment. *Vet Ophthalmol* 6: 15–17, 2003.

Bill A: Formation and drainage of aqueous humor in cats. *Exp Eye Res* 5: 185–190, 1966.

Del Sole MJ, Sande PH, Bernades JM, et al: Circadian rhythm of intraocular pressure in cats. *Vet Ophthalmol* 10: 155–161, 2007.

Kroll MM, Miller PE, Rodan R: Intraocular pressure measurements obtained as part of a comprehensive geriatric health examination from cats seven years of age or older. *J Am Vet Med Assoc* 219: 1406–1410, 2001.

Reviews

Brooks DE: Glaucomas in the dog and cat. *Vet Clin North Amer Small Anim Pract* 20: 775–797, 1990.

Dietrich U: Feline glaucomas. *Clin Tech Small Anim Pract* 20: 108–116, 2005.

Congenital

Brown A, Munger R, Peiffer RL: Congenital glaucoma and iridoschisis in a Siamese cat. *Vet Comp Ophthalmol* 4: 121–124, 1994.

Primary

Gelatt KN, Brooks DE, Samuelson DA: Comparative glaucomatology. I. The spontaneous glaucomas. *J Glaucoma* 7: 187–201, 1998.

Hampson EC, Smith RI, Bernays ME: Primary glaucoma in Burmese cats. *Aust Vet J* 2002: 80: 672–680.

Jacobi S, Dubielzig RR: Feline primary open angle glaucoma. *Vet Ophthalmol* 11: 162–165, 2008.

Trost K, Peiffer RL, Nell B: Goniodysgenesis associated with primary glaucoma in an adult European short-haired cat. *Vet Ophthalmol* 10 (Suppl): 3–7, 2007.

Aqueous Misdirection Syndrome

Czederpiltz JM, La Croix NC, van der Woerdt A, et al: Putative aqueous humor misdirection syndrome as a cause of glaucoma in cats: 32 cases (1997–2003). *J Am Vet Med Assoc* 227: 1434–1441, 2005.

Secondary

Blocker T, van der Woerdt A: The feline glaucomas: 82 cases (1995–1999). *Vet Ophthalmol* 4: 81–85, 2001.

Coop MC, Thomas JR: Bilateral glaucoma in the cat. *J Am Vet Med Assoc* 133: 369–370, 1958.

McCalla TL, Moore CP, Collier LL: Phacoclastic uveitis with secondary glaucoma in a cat. *Comp Anim Pract* 2: 13–17, 1988.

McLaughlin SA, Render JA, Brightman AH, et al: Intraocular findings in three dogs and one cat with chronic glaucoma. *J Am Vet Med Assoc* 191: 1443–1445, 1987.

Miller PE: Feline glaucoma, in Bonagura JD, Twedt DC (eds): *Kirk's Current Veterinary Therapy XIV*. St Louis, Saunders, 2009, pp 1207–1214.

Ridgeway MD, Brightman AH: Feline glaucoma: A retrospective study of 29 clinical cases. *J Am Anim Hosp Assoc* 25: 485–490, 1989.

Walde I, Rapp E: Feline glaucoma. Clinical and morphological aspects (a retrospective study of 38 cases). *Eur J Comp Anim Pract* 4: 87–105, 1993.

Wilcock BP, Peiffer RL Jr, Davidson MG: The causes of glaucoma in cats. *Vet Pathol* 27: 35–40, 1990.

Zahn GL, Miranda OC, Bito LZ: Steroid glaucoma: Corticosteroid-induced ocular hypertension in cats. *Curr Eye Res* 54: 211–218, 1992.

Diagnostics

Bentley E, Miller PE, Diehl KA: Use of high-resolution ultrasound as a diagnostic tool in veterinary ophthalmology. *J Am Vet Med Assoc* 223: 1617–1622, 2003.

Bryan GM: Tonometry in the dog and cat. *J Small Anim Pract* 6: 117–120, 1965.

Gelatt KN, Ladds PW: Gonioscopy in dogs and cats with glaucoma and ocular tumors. *J Small Anim Pract* 12: 105–117, 1971.

Rusanen E, Florin M, Hässig M, et al: Evalution of a rebound tonometer (Tonovet®) in clinically normal cat eyes. *Vet Ophthalmol* 13: 31–36, 2010.

Therapy

Bartoe JT, Davidson HJ, Horton MT, et al: The effects of bimatoprost and unoprostone isopropyl on the intraocular pressure of normal cats. *Vet Ophthalmol* 8: 247–252, 2005.

Bingaman DP, Lindley DM: Intraocular gentamicin and glaucoma: A retrospective study of 60 dog and cat eyes (1985–1993). *Vet Comp Ophthalmol* 4: 113–119, 1994.

Dietrich UM, Chandler MJ, Cooper T, et al: Effects of topical 2% dorzolamide hydrochloride alone and in combination with 0.5% timolol maleate on intraocular pressure in normal feline eyes. *Vet Ophthalmol* 10 (Suppl): 95–100, 2007.

Dugan SJ, Roberts SM, Severin GA: Systemic osmotherapy for ophthalmic disease in dogs and cats. *J Am Vet Med Assoc* 194: 115–118, 1989.

Gray HE, Willis AM, Morgan RV: Effects of topical administration of 1% brinzolamide on normal cat eyes. *Vet Ophthalmol* 6: 285–290, 2003.

Miller PE, Rhaesa SL: Effects of topical administration of 0.5% apraclonidine on intraocular pressure, pupil size, and heart rate of clinically normal cats. *Am J Vet Res* 57: 83–86, 1996.

Rainbow ME, Dziezyc J: Effects of twice daily application of 2% dorzolamide on intraocular pressure in normal cats. *Vet Ophthalmol* 6: 147–150, 2003.

Regnier A, Lemagne C, Ponchet A, et al.: Ocular effects of topical 0.03% bimatoprost solution in normotensive feline eyes. *Vet Ophthalmol* 9: 39–43, 2006.

Studer ME, Martin CL, Stiles J: Effects of 0.005% latanoprost solution on intraocular pressure in healthy dogs and cats. *Am J Vet Res* 61: 1220–1224, 2000.

Wilkie DA, Latimer CA: Effects of topical administration of timolol maleate on intraocular pressure and pupil size in cats. *Am J Vet Res* 52: 436–440, 1991.

Wilkie DA, Latimer CA: Effects of topical administration of 2.0% pilocarpine on intraocular pressure and pupil size in cats. *Am J Vet Res* 52: 441–444, 1991.

Willis AM: Ocular hypotensive drugs. *Vet Clin North Am Small Anim Pract* 34: 755–776, 2004.

LENS

Anomalies

Aguirre GD, Bistner SI: Microphakia with lenticular luxation and subluxation in cats. *Vet Med Small Anim Clin* 68: 498–500, 1973.

Molleda J, Martin E: Microphakia associated with lens luxation in the cat. *J Am Anim Hosp Assoc* 31: 209–212, 1995.

Peiffer RL: Bilateral congenital aphakia and retinal detachment in a cat. *J Am Anim Hosp Assoc* 18: 128–130, 1982.

Peiffer RL: Keratolenticular dysgenesis in a kitten. *J Am Vet Med Assoc* 182: 1242–1243, 1983.

Cataract

Gilger BC, Davidson MG, Howard PB: Keratometry, ultrasonic biometry, and prediction of intraocular lens power in the feline eye. *Am J Vet Res* 59: 131–134, 1998.

Gilger BC, Davidson MG, Colitz CM: Experimental implantation of posterior chamber prototype intraocular lenses for the feline eye. *Am J Vet Res* 59: 1339–1343, 1998.

Peiffer RL, Gelatt KN: Cataracts in the cat. *Feline Pract* 4: 34–38, 1974.

Peiffer RL, Gelatt KN: Congenital cataracts in a Persian kitten. *Vet Med Small Anim Clin* 70: 1334–1335, 1975.

Rubin LF: Hereditary cataract in Himalayan cats. *Feline Pract* 16: 14–15, 1986.

Sapienza JS: Feline lens disorders. *Clin Tech Small Anim Pract* 20: 102–107, 2005.

Schwink K: Posterior nuclear cataracts in two Birman kittens. *Feline Pract* 16: 31–33, 1986.

Williams DL, Heath MF: Prevalence of feline cataract: results of a cross-sectional study of 2000 normal animals, 50 cats with diabetes and one hundred cats following dehydrational crises. *Vet Ophthalmol* 9: 341–349, 2006.

Nutritional

Remillard RL, Pickett JP, Thatcher CD, et al: Comparison of kittens fed queen's milk with those fed milk replacers. *Am J Vet Res* 54: 901–907, 1993.

Metabolic

Richter M, Guscetti F: Aldose reductase activity and glucose-related opacities in incubated lenses from dogs and cats. *Am J Vet Res* 63: 1591–1597, 2002.

Stiles J: Cataracts in a kitten with nutritional secondary hyperparathyroidism. *Prog Vet Comp Ophthalmol* 1: 296–298, 1991.

Thoresen S, Bjerkas E: Diabetes mellitus and bilateral cataracts in a kitten. *J Feline Med Surg* 4: 115–122, 2002.

Luxation

Curtis R: Lens luxation in the dog and cat. *Vet Clin North Am Small Anim Pract* 20: 755–773, 1990.

Olivero DK, Riis RC, Dutton AG, et al: Feline lens displacement: A retrospective analysis of 345 cases. *Prog Vet Comp Ophthalmol* 1: 239–244, 1991.

Payen G, Hänninen RL, Mazzucchelli S, et al: Lens instability in ten related cats: Clinical and genetic considerations. *J Small Anim Pract* 52: 402–410, 2011.

VITREOUS

Allgoewer I, Pfefferkorn B: Persistent hyperplastic tunica vasculosa lentis and persistent hyperplastic primary vitreous (PHTVL/PHPV) in two cats. *Vet Ophthalmol* 4: 161–164, 2001.

Leon A: Diseases of the vitreous in the dog and cat. *J Small Anim Pract* 29: 448–461, 1988.

RETINA

Anatomy/Physiology

Blake R, Bellhorn RW: Visual acuity in cats with central retinal lesions. *Vision Res* 18: 15–18, 1978.

De Schaepdrijver L, Simoens P, Lauwers H: Morphologic and fluorangiographic study of the feline retina. *Vet Comp Ophthalmol* 7: 216–225, 1997.

Donovan A: The postnatal development of the cat retina. *Exp Eye Res* 5: 249–254, 1966.

Henkind P: The retinal vascular system of the domestic cat. *Exp Eye Res* 5: 10–20, 1966.

Johnson BW: Congenitally abnormal visual pathways of Siamese cats. *Comp Cont Educ Vet* 13: 374–377, 1991.

Kalil RE, Jhaveri SR, Richards W: Anomalous retinal pathways in the Siamese cat: An inadequate substrate for normal binocular vision. *Science* 174: 302–305, 1971.

Ollivier FJ, Samuelson DA, Brooks DE, et al: Comparative morphology of the tapetum lucidum (among selected species). *Vet Ophthalmol* 7: 11–22, 2004.

Steinberg R, Reid M, Lacy P: The distribution of rods and cones in the retina of the cat (*Felis domesticus*). *J Comp Neurol* 148: 229–248, 1973.

Congenital

Albert DM, Lahav M, Colby ED, et al: Retinal neoplasia and dysplasia. I. Induction by feline leukemia virus. *Invest Ophthalmol Vis Sci* 16: 325–337, 1977.

Percy DH, Scott FW, Albert DM: Retinal dysplasia due to feline panleukopenia virus infection. *J Am Vet Med Assoc* 167: 935–937, 1975.

MacMillan AD: Retinal dysplasia in the dog and cat. *Vet Clin North Am Small Anim Pract* 10: 411–415, 1980.

Wen GY, Wisniewski HM, Sturman JA: Hereditary abnormality in tapetum lucidum of the Siamese cat: A histochemical and quantitative study. *Histochemistry* 75: 1–9, 1982.

Chorioretinitis (See Also Anterior Uveitis)

Toxoplasmosis

Campbell LH: Toxoplasma retinitis in a cat. *Feline Pract* 4: 36–39, 1974.

Ophthalmomyiasis

Brooks DE, Wolf ED, Merideth RE: Ophthalmomyiasis interna in two cats. *J Am Anim Hosp Assoc* 20: 157–160, 1984.

Gwin RM: Ophthalmomyiasis interna posterior in two cats and a dog. *J Am Anim Hosp Assoc* 20: 481–486, 1984.

Kaswan R, Martin C: Ophthalmomyiasis in a dog and cat. *Canine Pract* 11: 28–34, 1984.

Wyman M, Starkey R, Weisbrode S, et al: Ophthalmomyiasis (interna posterior) of the posterior segment and central nervous system myiasis: *Cuterebra spp* in a cat. *Vet Ophthalmol* 8: 77–80, 2005.

Hypertensive Retinopathy

Belew AM, Barlett T, Brown SA: Evaluation of the white-coat effect in cats. *J Vet Intern Med* 13: 134–142, 1999.

Bodey AR, Sansom J: Epidemiological study of blood pressure in domestic cats. *J Small Anim Pract* 39: 567–573, 1998.

Crispin SM, Mould JR: Systemic hypertensive disease and the feline fundus. *Vet Ophthalmol* 4: 131–140, 2001.

Dukes J: Hypertension: A review of the mechanisms, manifestations and management. *J Small Anim Pract* 33: 119–129, 1992.

Elliott J, Barber PJ, Syme HM, et al: Feline hypertension: clinical findings and response to antihypertensive treatment in 30 cases. *J Small Anim Pract* 42: 122–129, 2001.

Haberman CE, Morgan JD, Kang CW, et al: Evaluation of Dopper ultrasonic and oscillometric methods of indirect blood pressure measurement in cats. *Internat J Appl Res Vet Med* 2: 279–289, 2004.

Kobayashi DL, Peterson ME, Graves TK, et al: Hypertension in cats with chronic renal failure or hyperthyroidism. *J Vet Intern Med* 4: 58–62, 1990.

Komaromy AM, Andrew SE, Denis HM, et al: Hypertensive retinopathy and choroidopathy in a cat. *Vet Ophthalmol* 7: 3–9, 2004.

Lane IF, Roberts SM, Lappin MR: Ocular manifestations of vascular disease: Hypertension, hyperviscosity and hyperlipidemia. *J Am Anim Hosp Assoc* 29: 28–36, 1993.

Littman MP: Spontaneous systemic hypertension in 24 cats. *J Vet Intern Med* 8: 79–86, 1994.

Maggio F, de Francesco TC, Atkins CE, et al: Ocular lesions associated with systemic hypertension in cats: 69 cases (1985–1998). *J Am Vet Med Assoc* 217: 695–702, 2000.

Mathur S, Syme H, Brown CA, et al: Effects of the calcium channel antagonist amlodipine in cats with surgically induced hypertensive renal insufficiency. *Am J Vet Res* 63: 833–839, 2002.

Morgan RV: Systemic hypertension in four cats: Ocular and medical findings. *J Am Anim Hosp Assoc* 22: 615–621, 1986.

Sansom J, Barnett KC, Dunn KA, et al: Ocular disease associated with hypertension in 16 cats. *J Small Anim Pract* 35: 604–611, 1994.

Sansom J, Rogers K, Wood JL: Blood pressure assessment in healthy cats and cats with hypertensive retinopathy. *Am J Vet Res* 65: 245–252, 2004.

Stiles J, Polzin DJ, Bistner SI: The prevalence of retinopathy in cats with systemic hypertension and chronic retinal failure or hyperthyroidism. *J Am Anim Hosp Assoc* 30: 564–572, 1994.

Synder PS: Amlodipine: A randomized, blinded clinical trial of 9 cats with systemic hypertension. *J Vet Intern Med* 12: 157–162, 1998.

Turner JL, Brogdon JD, Lees GE, et al: Idiopathic hypertension in a cat with secondary hypertensive retinopathy associated with a high-salt diet. *J Am Anim Hosp Assoc* 26: 647–651, 1990.

Retinal Detachment

Anderson DH, Guerin CJ, Erikson PA, et al: Morphological recovery in the reattached retina. *Invest Ophthalmol Vis Sci* 27: 168–183, 1986.

Anderson DH, Stern WH, Fisher SK, et al: Retinal detachment in the cat: The pigment epithelial-photoreceptor interface. *Invest Ophthalmol Vis Sci* 24: 906–926, 1983.

Erickson PA, Fisher SK, Anderson DH, et al: Retinal detachment in the cat: the outer nuclear and outer plexiform layers. *Invest Ophthalmol Vis Sci* 24: 927–942, 1983.

Formston C: Retinal detachment and bovine tuberculosis in cats. *J Small Anim Pract* 35:5–8, 1994.

Lombard CW, Twitchell MJ: Tetralogy of fallot, persistent left cranial vena cava, and retinal detachment in a cat. *J Am Anim Hosp Assoc* 14: 624–630, 1978.

Roberts SR: Detachment of the retina in animals. *J Am Vet Med Assoc* 135: 423–432, 1959.

Retinopathy

Reviews

Barnett KC, Curtis R, Millichamp NJ: The differential diagnosis of retinal degeneration in the dog and cat. *J Small Anim Pract* 663–673, 1983.

Curtis R: Retinal diseases in the dog and cat: An overview and update. *J Small Anim Pract* 29: 397–415, 1988.

Retinal folds

MacMillan AD: Acquired retinal folds in the cat. *J Am Vet Med Assoc* 168: 1015–1020, 1976.

Fluoroquinolone

Ford MM, Dubielzig RR, Giuliano EA, et al: Ocular and systemic manifestations after oral administration of a high dose of enrofloxacin in cats. *Am J Vet Res* 68: 190–202, 2007.

Gelatt KN, van der Woerdt A, Ketring KL, et al: Enrofloxacin-associated retinal degeneration in cats. *Vet Ophthalmol* 4: 99–106, 2001.

Wiebe V, Hamilton P: Fluoroquinolone-induced retinal degeneration in cats. *J Am Vet Med Assoc* 221: 1568–1571, 2002.

Miscellaneous toxicities

Barclay SM, Riis RC: Retinal detachment and reattachment associated with ethylene glycol intoxication in a cat. *J Am Anim Hosp Assoc* 15: 719–724, 1979.

Schaller J, Wyman M, Weisbrode S, et al: Induction of retinal degeneration in cats by methylnitrosurea and ketamine hydrochloride. *Vet Pathol* 18: 239–247, 1981.

Feline central retinal degeneration (FCRD)

Aguirre GD: Retinal degeneration associated with the feeding of dog foods to cats. *J Am Vet Med Assoc* 172: 791–796, 1978.

Anderson PA, Baker DH, Corbin JE, et al: Biochemical lesions associated with taurine deficiency in the cat. *J Anim Sci* 49: 1227–1234, 1979.

Barnett KC, Burger IH: Taurine deficiency retinopathy in the cat. *J Small Anim Pract* 21: 521–534, 1980.

Bedford PGC: Feline central retinal degeneration in the United Kingdom. *Vet Rec* 112: 456–457, 1983.

Bellhorn RW, Aguirre GD, Bellhorn MB: Feline central retinal degeneration. *Invest Ophthalmol Vis Sci* 13: 608–616, 1974.

Bellhorn RW, Fischer CA: Feline central retinal degeneration. *J Am Vet Med Assoc* 157: 842–849, 1970.

Blake R, Bellhorn RW: Visual acuity in cats with central retinal lesions. *Exp Eye Res* 18: 15–18, 1978.

Berson EL, Hayes KC, Rabin AR, et al: Retinal degeneration in cats fed casein. II. Supplementation with methionine, cysteine or taurine. *Invest Ophthalmol Vis Sci* 15: 52–58, 1976.

da Costa P, Hoskins J: The role of taurine in cats: Current concepts. *Compend Cont Educ Vet* 12: 1235–1240, 1990.

Hayes KC, Carey RE, Schmidt SY: Retinal degeneration associated with taurine deficiency in the cat. *Science* 188: 949–951, 1975.

Hayes KC, Rabin AR, Berson EL: An ultrastructural study of nutritionally induced and reversed retinal degeneration in cats. *Am J Pathol* 78: 505–524, 1975.

Hickman MA: Bioavailability of taurine for cats. *Compend Cont Educ Vet* 22: 33–35, 2000.

Leon A, Levick WR, Sarossy MG: Lesion topography and new histological features in feline taurine deficiency retinopathy. *Exp Eye Res* 61: 731–741, 1995.

Morris ML: Feline degenerative retinopathy. *Cornell Vet* 55: 295–308, 1965.

Rabin A, Hayes K, Berson E: Cone and rod responses in nutritionally-induced retinal degeneration in the cat. *Invest Ophthalmol Vis Sci* 12: 694–704, 1973.

Ricketts J: Feline central retinal degeneration in the domestic cat. *J Small Anim Pract* 24: 221–227, 1983.

Schmidt SY, Berson EL, Hayes KC: Retinal degeneration in cats fed casein. I. Taurine deficiency. *Invest Ophthalmol Vis Sci* 15: 47–52, 1976.

Schmidt SY, Berson EL, Watson G, et al: Retinal degeneration in cats fed casein. III. Taurine deficiency and ERG amplitudes. *Invest Ophthalmol Vis Sci* 16: 673–678, 1977.

Scott PP, Greaves JP, Scott MG: Nutritional blindness in the cat. *Exp Eye Res* 3: 357–364, 1964.

Wen GY, Sturman JA, Wisniewski HM, et al: Tapetum disorganization in taurine-depleted cats. *Invest Ophthalmol Vis Sci* 18: 1200–1206, 1979.

Progressive retinal atrophy

Anderson RE, Maude MB, Nilsson SEG, et al: Plasma lipid abnormalities in the Abyssinian cat with a hereditary rod-cone degeneration. *Exp Eye Res* 53: 415–417, 1991.

Barnett KC: Retinal atrophy. *Vet Rec* 77: 1543–1560, 1965.

Barnett KC: Progressive retinal atrophy in the Abyssinian cat. *J Small Anim Pract* 23: 763–766, 1982.

Barnett KC, Curtis R: Autosomal dominant progressive retinal atrophy in Abyssinian cats. *J Hered* 76: 168–170, 1985.

Bedford PGC: Control of inherited retinal degeneration in dogs and cats in the United Kingdom. *J Small Anim Pract* 30: 172–177, 1989.

Carlile JL: Feline retinal atrophy. *Vet Rec* 108: 311, 1981.

Carlile JL, Carrington SD, Bedford PGC: Six cases of progressive retinal atrophy in Abyssinian cats. *J Small Anim Pract* 25: 415–420, 1984.

Chong NH, Alexander RA, Barnett KC, et al: An immunohistochemical study of an autosomal dominant feline rod/cone dysplasia (*rdy* cats). *Exp Eye Res* 68: 51–57, 1999.

Curtis R, Barnett KC, Leon A: An early-onset retinal dystrophy with dominant inheritance in the Abyssinian cat: Clinical and pathological findings. *Invest Ophthalmol Vis Sci* 28: 131–139, 1987.

Derwent JJ, Padnick-Silver L, McRipley M, et al: The electroretinogram components in Abyssinian cats with hereditary retinal degeneration. *Invest Ophthalmol Vis Sci* 47: 3673–3682, 2006.

Ehinger B, Narfstrom K, Nilsson SE, et al: Photoreceptor degeneration and loss of immunoreactive GABA in the Abyssinian cat retina. *Exp Eye Res* 52: 17–25, 1991.

Ekesten B, Narfström K: Abnormal dark-adapted ERG in cats heterozygous for a recessively inherited rod-cone degeneration. *Vet Ophthalmol* 7: 63–67, 2004.

Giuliano EA, van der Woerdt A: Feline retinal degeneration: clinical experience and new findings (1994–1997). *J Am Anim Hosp Assoc* 35: 511–514, 1999.

Gorin MB, To AC, Narfström K: Sequence analysis and exclusion of phosducin as the gene for the recessive retinal degeneration of the Abyssinian cat. *Biochem Biophys Acta* 1260: 323–327, 1995.

Gould DJ, Sargan DR: Autosomal dominant retinal dystrophy (*rdy*) in Abyssinian cats: Exclusion of PDE6G and ROM1 and likely exclusion of rhodopsin as candidate genes. *Anim Genet* 33: 436–440, 2002.

Hyman JA, Vaegan MA, Lei B, et al: Electrophysiologic differentiation of homozygous and heterozygous Abyssinian-crossbred cats with late-onset hereditary retinal degeneration. *Am J Vet Res* 66: 1914–1921, 2005.

Jacobson SG, Kemp CM, Narfström K, et al: Rhodopsin levels and rod-mediated function in Abyssinian cats with hereditary retinal degeneration. *Exp Eye Res* 49: 843–852, 1989.

Kelly D, Lewis D: Rapidly progressive diffuse retinal degeneration in a kitten. *J Small Anim Pract* 26: 317–322, 1985.

Leon A, Curtis R: Autosomal dominant rod-cone dysplasia in the *rdy* cat. 1. Light and electron microscopic findings. *Exp Eye Res* 51: 361–381, 1990.

Leon A, Hussain AA, Curtis R: Autosomal dominant rod-cone dysplasia in the rdy cat. 2. Electrophysiological findings. *Exp Eye Res* 53: 489–502, 1991.

May CA, Narfstrom K: Choroidal microcirculation in Abyssinian cats with hereditary rod-cone degeneration. *Exp Eye Res* 86: 537–540, 2008.

May CA, Lutjen-Drecoll E, Narfstrom K: Morphological changes in the anterior segment of the Abyssinian cat eye with hereditary rod-cone degeneration. *Curr Eye Res* 30: 855–862, 2005.

Menotti-Raymond M, David VA, Pflueger S, et al: Widespread retinal degenerative disease mutation (*rdAc*) discovered among a larger number of popular cat breeds. *Vet J* 186: 32–38, 2010.

Menotti-Raymond M, David VA, Schäffer AA, et al: Mutation in CEP290 discovered for cat model of human retinal degeneration. *J Hered* 98: 211–220, 2007.

Morris M: Feline degenerative retinopathy. *Cornell Vet* 60: 295–308, 1965.

Narfstrom K: Hereditary progressive retinal atrophy in the Abyssinian cat. *J Hered* 74: 273–276, 1983.

Narfstrom K: Progressive retinal atrophy in the Abyssinian cat. *Clinical characterisics. Invest Ophthalmol Vis Sci* 26: 193–200, 1985.

Narfström K, David V, Jarret O, et al: Retinal degeneration in the Abyssinian and Somali cat (*rdAc*): Correlation between genotype and phenotype and *rdAc* allele frequency in two continents. *Vet Ophthalmol* 12: 285–291, 2009.

Narfström K, Ehinger B, Bruun A: Immunohistochemical studies of cone photoreceptors and cells of the inner retina in feline rod-cone degeneration. *Vet Ophthalmol* 4: 141–145, 2001.

Narfström K, Nilsson SE: Hereditary retinal degeneration in the Abyssinian cat: correlation of ophthalmoscopic and electroretinographic findings. *Doc Ophthalmol* 60: 183–187, 1985.

Narfström K, Nilsson SE: Progressive retinal atrophy in the Abyssinian cat. Electron microscopy. *Invest Ophthalmol Vis Sci* 27: 1569–1576, 1986.

Narfström K, Nilsson SE: Morphological findings during retinal development and maturation in hereditary rod-cone degeneration in Abyssinian cats. *Exp Eye Res* 49: 611–628, 1989.

Narfström KL, Nilsson SE, Andersson BE: Progressive retinal atrophy in the Abyssinian cat: Studies of the DC-recorded electroretinogram and the standing potential of the eye. *Br J Ophthalmol* 69: 618–623, 1985.

Padnick-Silver L, Kang Derwent JJ, Giuliano E, et al: Retinal oxygenation and oxygen metabolism in Abyssinian cats with a hereditary retinal degeneration. *Invest Ophthalmol Vis Sci* 47: 3683–3689, 2006.

Rah H, Maggs DJ, Blankenship TN, et al: Early-onset, autosomal recessive, progressive retinal atrophy in Persian cats. *Invest Ophthalmol Vis Sci* 46: 1742–1747, 2005.

Rubin LF: Atrophy of rods and cones in the cat retina. *J Am Vet Med Assoc* 142: 1415–1420, 1963.

Rubin LF, Lipton DE: Retinal degeneration in kittens. *J Am Vet Med Assoc* 62: 467–469, 1973.

Souri E: Observations of feline retinal degenerations. *Vet Med Small Anim Clin* 67: 983–986, 1972.

Thompson S, Whiting REH, Kardon RH, et al: Effects of hereditary retinal degeneration due to a CEP290 mutation on the feline pupillary light reflex. *Vet Ophthalmol* 13: 151–157, 2010.

West-Hyde L, Buyukmihci N: Photoreceptor degeneration in a family of cats. *J Am Vet Med Assoc* 181: 243–247, 1982.

Wiggert B, van Veen T, Kutty G, et al: An early decrease in interphotoreceptor retinoid-binding protein gene expression in Abyssinian cats homozygous for hereditary rod-cone degeneration. *Cell Tissue Res* 278: 291–298, 1994.

Other retinal degenerations

Barone G, Foureman P, deLahunta A: Adult-onset cerebellar cortical abiotrophy and retinal degeneration in a domestic short-hair cat. *J Am Anim Hosp Assoc* 38: 51–54, 2002.

Valle D, Boison A, Jezyk P, et al: Gyrate atrophy of the choroid and retina in a cat. *Invest Ophthal Vis Sci* 20: 251–254, 1981.

Chediak-Higashi syndrome

Creel D, Collier LL, Leventhal AG, et al: Abnormal retinal projections in cats with the Chédiak-Higashi syndrome. *Invest Ophthalmol Vis Sci* 23: 798–801, 1982.

Collier LL, King EJ, Prieur DJ: Aberrant melanosome development in the retinal pigment epithelium of cats with Chédiak-Higashi syndrome. *Exp Eye Res* 41: 305–311, 1985.

Collier LL, King EJ, Prieur DJ: Tapetal degeneration in cats with Chediak-Higashi syndrome. *Curr Eye Res* 4: 767–773, 1985.

Collier LL, Prieur DJ, King EJ: Ocular melanin pigmentation anomalies in cats, cattle, mink, and mice with Chédiak-Higashi syndrome: Histologic observations. *Curr Eye Res* 3: 1241–1251, 1984.

Storage Diseases

Skelly BJ, Franklin RJ: Recognition and diagnosis of lysosomal storage diseases in the cat and dog. *J Vet Intern Med* 16: 133–141, 2002.

Metabolic/Vascular Changes

Lipemia retinalis

Crispin SM: Ocular manifestations of hyperlipoproteinanemia. *J Small Anim Pract* 34: 500–506, 1993.

Jones BR, Wallace A, Harding DR, et al: Occurrence of idiopathic, familial hyperchylomicronaemia in a cat. *Vet Rec* 112: 543–547, 1983.

Wyman M, McKissick GE: Lipemia retinalis in a dog and cat: case reports. *J Am Anim Hosp Assoc* 9: 288–291, 1973.

Hyperviscosity syndrome

Forrester SD, Greco DS, Relford RL: Serum hyperviscosity syndrome associated with multiple myeloma in two cats. *J Am Vet Med Assoc* 200: 79–82, 1992.

Foster ES, Lothrop CD: Polycythemia vera in a cat with cardiac hypertrophy. *J Am Vet Med Assoc* 192: 1736–1738, 1988.

Hribernik TN, Barta O, Gaunt SD, et al: Serum hyperviscosity syndrome associated with IgG myeloma in a cat. *J Am Anim Hosp Assoc* 181: 169–170, 1982.

Williams DA, Goldschmidt MH: Hyperviscosity syndrome with IgM monoclonal gammopathy and hepatic plasmacytoid lymphosarcoma. *J Small Anim Pract* 23: 311–323, 1982.

Diabetic retinopathy

Herrtage ME, Barnett KC, MacDougall DF: Diabetic retinopathy in a cat with megestrol acetate-induced diabetes. *J Small Anim Pract* 26: 595–601, 1985.

Retinal hemorrhage

Fischer CA: Retinopathy in anemic cats. *J Am Vet Med Assoc* 156: 1415–1427, 1970.

Neoplasia

Cassotis NJ, Dubielzig RR, Gilger BC, et al: Angioinvasive pulmonary carcinoma with posterior segment metastasis in four cats. *Vet Ophthalmol* 2: 125–131, 1999.

Cook CS, Peiffer RL, Stine PE: Metastatic ocular squamous cell carcinoma in a cat. *J Am Vet Med Assoc* 185: 1547–1549, 1984.

Semin MO, Serra F, Make V, et al: Choroidal melanocytoma in a cat. *Vet Ophthalmol* 14: 205–208, 2011.

Williams DL, Goldschmidt MH: Hyperviscosity syndrome with IgM monoclonal gammopathy and hepatic plasmacytoid lymphosarcoma in a cat. *J Small Anim Pract* 23: 311–323, 1982.

OPTIC NERVE

Anatomy

Ng AY, Stone J: The optic nerve of the cat: Appearance and loss of axons during normal development. *Brain Res* 281: 263–271, 1982.

Radius RL, Bade B: The anatomy at the lamina cribrosa in the normal cat eye. *Arch Ophthalmol* 100: 1658–1660, 1982.

Coloboma

Martin C, Stiles J, Willis M: Feline colobomatous syndrome. *Vet Comp Ophthalmol* 7: 39–43, 1997.

Hypoplasia

Barnett K, Grimes T: Bilateral aplasia of the optic nerve in a cat. *Br J Ophthalmol* 57: 663–667, 1974.

Optic Neuritis/Neuropathy

Nell B: Optic neuritis in dogs and cats. *Vet Clin North Am Small Anim Pract* 38: 403–415, 2008.

Stiles J, Buyukmihci NC, Hacker DV, et al: Blindness from damage to the optic chiasm [letter to editor]. *J Am Vet Med Assoc* 202: 1192, 1993.

CENTRAL BLINDNESS

Davidson MG, Nasisse MP, Breitschwerdt EB, et al: Acute blindness associated with intracranial tumors in dogs and cats: Eight cases (1984–1989). *J Am Vet Med Assoc* 199: 755–758, 1991.

Seruca C, Rodenas S, Leiva M, et al: Acute postretinal blindness: Ophthalmologic, neurologic, and magnetic resonance imaging findings in dogs and cats (seven cases). *Vet Ophthalmol* 13: 307–314, 2010.

MISCELLANEOUS

Ocular Anomalies/Hereditary Diseases

Barnett KC: Inherited eye disease in the dog and cat. *J Small Anim Pract* 29: 462–475, 1988.

Cook CS: Embryogenesis of congenital eye malformations. *Vet Comp Ophthalmol* 5: 109–123, 1995.

Glaze MB: Congenital and hereditary ocular abnormalities in cats. *Clin Tech Small Anim Pract* 20: 74–82, 2005.

Narfström K: Hereditary and congenital ocular disease in the cat. *J Feline Med Surg* 1: 135–141, 1999.

Peiffer RL: Inherited ocular diseases of the dog and cat. *Compend Cont Educ Vet* 4: 154–164, 1982.

Priester WA: Congenital ocular defects in cattle, horses, cats, and dogs. *J Am Vet Med Assoc* 160: 1504–1511, 1972.

Saperstein G, Harris S, Leipold HW: Congenital defects in domestic cats. *Feline Pract* 6: 18–27, 1976.

Wilcock B: Ocular anomalies, in Peiffer RL (ed): Comparative Ophthalmic Pathology. Springfield, CC Thomas, 1983, pp 3–46.

Ocular Emergencies

Giuliano EA: Feline ocular emergencies. *Clin Tech Small Anim Pract* 20: 135–141, 2005.

Jurk IR, Thibodeau MS, Whitney K, et al: Acute vision loss after general anesthesia in a cat. *Vet Ophthalmol* 4: 155–158, 2001.

Systemic Disease-Related Images

The following index is to aid in identifying ocular conditions related to specific systemic diseases.